Finding the Wheel's Hub

Tales and thoughts from the endurance athletic lifestyle

D0067695

Scott Tinley

Published by The Trimarket Company, Palo Alto, California, USA

Library of Congress Cataloging-in-Publication Data

Tinley, Scott.
    Finding the wheel's hub : tales and thoughts from the endurance athletic lifestyle /
    Scott Tinley.
            p.   cm.
    ISBN 0-9634568-5-7
        1. Triathlon–Anecdotes.   2. Physical fitness–Psychological aspects.
    3. Athletes–Anecdotes.   I. Title.
    GV342.22.T56   1995
    796.4' 07–dc20
                                                                        95-128
                                                                        CIP

Published by: The Trimarket Company, P. O. Box 60871, Palo Alto, California 94306

Photos: David Epperson (front cover), Tony Svensson (back cover)
Cover design: Trimarket and Pixelmedia
Color separations: Pixelmedia

Production notes: This book was created using FrameMaker® from Frame Technology Corporation on a PowerBook® Duo and Power Macintosh® computers from Apple Computer, Inc. The artwork was produced using Adobe Illustrator® and the photos manipulated using Adobe Photoshop® from Adobe Systems, Inc.

Printed in the United States of America

                                                            ISBN 0-9634568-5-7
                                    Library of Congress Catalog Card Number: 95-128

Scott Tinley clearly and concisely points the way. *Finding the Wheel's Hub* blends philosophical thinking with practical experience– a book competitors from Wall Street to the race car track can relate to.

Danny Sullivan
Indianapolis 500 winner

This book was written by Scott Tinley over a period of many years. Some of this material has been published in *Triathlete, Inside Triathlon, Triathlon Sports Australia* and other sports related publications.

The Publisher

A special thanks to Lauren Rusk of Stanford University, patient linguist and copy editor of the previously unpublished material.

To Ruthie,

and the memory of her son
and to mothers of sons
everywhere

Preface

In the process of compiling this collection of articles, a few things became obvious. First, the articles were written over a period of eight years for publications such as *Triathlete, Inside Triathlon, Triathlon Sports Australia* and the occasional general fitness magazine. From a standpoint of style and readability, I was hoping that they improved. In fact, that is why many of the early pieces didn't make the cut. Their sophomoric nature more than hinted that I was a professional athlete without any formal training in writing. A million words later, I am still a professional athlete without formal training. But I enjoy the writing, so I continue.

It also became obvious that beyond telling a story or offering a tip, writing these articles was a type of self-cleansing process. If I wrote it down, it became clearer–whether trying to explain gear ratios (which I still can't) or how to sneak into the awards banquet, or poking fun at Kenny Souza's bikini shorts. On paper, the words had a place and meaning, for me at least.

I would sit up late at night when the house was quiet and everyone asleep, the lights down low. Armed with early Dylan CDs, I'd get out my yellow legal pad and just go. Given the scenario and the freedom to explore, rather than explain hill climbing techniques, I'm going to sit you down, pour you a beer and tell you about the time in 1983 when Scott Molina and I purposely tied for first place so we would both get a victory bonus from our sponsors. For the opportunity to tell these stories, I am very grateful.

I am also grateful to Bill Katovsky for my first assignment to pen a funky Q&A column in the early days of *Triathlete* and to Mike Plant who coauthored my first book and who said one day after reading something I wrote, "Write like you feel, like you're talking to a friend. Not like you know what you're doing, because you don't"–he was right. In addition, to Harold Johnson for "cleaning up" my worst pieces; Jean Claude Garot for keeping me on the back page all these years; Ken McAlpine, who did a heroic job on our second book and showed me how to apply professionalism to the trade; Dolores and Annette at Tinley for typing my hieroglyphics; all the players in my career who provided the elements and backdrop for my memories and tales; and especially to my wife VT, for never laughing at me (among other things), I thank you.

You see, my involvement in this sport is, like the book, a collection of experiences–good and bad, ugly and beautiful. Early on, I had to decide on the depth of my commitment. And early on, I realized that the lifestyle this profession provides could be one rich in taste and variety, but would necessitate a precarious balance between preparation, competition, professionalism, support systems and the real world of family, friends and paying the rent.

There is always a decision that requires thought, the act of weighing sides. And many times, I would roll the dice–chase the new race in some third world country, try the latest set of race wheels, call bullshit on some political maneuvering–hoping to find meaning.

Occasionally, some readers misunderstood my intentions. That's OK, though. Most of my articles were never meant to be commercially viable. Without limits or restrictions from editors and with little if any editing of my own, they took on more of a diary-like form rather than that of the safe and sedate "How To." Indeed, not being one to wear my heart on my sleeve, I often say things in these articles that I shy away from in conversation.

But I always figure that you only go around once and that second chances are rare. Rarer still are those fleeting moments when what we do makes sense, where the pieces of the puzzle fit.

I think we have a duty to ourselves to at least try to "figure it out." Sort of like looking for the wheel's hub, the center of a design where all the peripheral elements attach. For many people, this hub is family, spouse, hometown or career. As it should be. For an endurance athlete, the hub is often athletic movement itself.

It is the process, not the end result, that shapes us and allows us to continue our journey, rolling on, to whatever it is we seek.

There is little I would change.

Finding the Wheel's Hub

Contents

Chapter 1

What a Long, Strange Trip It's Been

Before we even arrived on the scene, you could feel the tragedy, sense the carnage. Sometimes it's like that. You know shit's going to hit the fan even before it does.

It was 1980. I was 24, going on 40, earning minimum wage while enjoying a street level education not included in the 60s suburban package. My job as a big city paramedic was a situational roller coaster, laden with urgency, stress and death. It is still the best gig I ever had.

Arriving at a multiple injury accident, rubbing three in the morning sleep from my eyes, the sight of half a dozen guys my age scattered over 200 yards was wild. We were the first responder to a truck that had rolled over with five guys in the bed, squashing two and seriously injuring the other three. In a triage situation where emergency resources are temporarily limited, you can only treat those who have the best chance for survival. You go about your work quietly, without emotion, splicing speed with efficiency, silently praying for help. But afterward, you always wonder if you were good enough, if you could have made a bigger difference. My partner and I did the best we could that night, but it's always overwhelming to have chosen who lives and who doesn't. The next day I became a triathlete.

Working 24 hour shifts with several days off in a row, I'd fill those days and blow off tension by swimming, cycling and running. This time, I felt the need to go at it all day. And though there were then no professional opportunities in triathlon, after a full day, I knew I could adapt to and enjoy a lifestyle that had at its core swimming, biking and running. Everything was different after that.

Almost fifteen years, a few hundred races and a million airline miles later, I regret very little of what I have done, least of all having chosen this particular career track. It's an incredible luxury to have work that can be a springboard to other areas of exploration. Too many people have jobs that lock them into a controlled, repetitive environment. But that's the way it is. You gotta eat and you need a roof over your head. To be able to experience new places, meet people from other countries and jump into situations that seem intimidating, but end up vastly rewarding–that's neat.

I've had the opportunity to swim with dolphins in Australia, climb a volcano in Chile, sleep in a hammock on Guam and run through the bowels of Harlem, New York–all because I'm a triathlete. I've also had a gun drawn on me, broken a bone or two, spent countless hours in smoky airplanes and cheap hotel rooms, and have been so sore and tired I couldn't get out of bed–all because I'm a triathlete.

But regardless of your job title, you too can fill up your memory banks with exotic, far-out experiences by simply opening your eyes and ears. Take a good look at the big picture *and* the little nuances that at first seem mundane, but upon further inspection reveal that what makes life interesting is not on the shelf, but under the rock.

Beyond the benefit of seeing more clearly, it can become obvious, if you strive, as they say, to "reach your goal," that what you achieve is not the golden fleece. Reaching your goal is great, but then what? Another goal? And then another? Soon it becomes clear that it's the process, the journey, the search that counts.

There is no finish line, just a series of mile markers. We all reach the final goal soon enough. Especially those who shun seatbelts.

GUIDANCE INTANGIBLE

Like many things in life, you never fully realize the effect that some-one or something has on you until you yourself are in a position to cause a similar catalyst. This theory is most often substantiated when a child grows up to be an adult, has his or her children, and realizes that what their parents did in raising them had rhyme and reason, or lack thereof. It's like Mark Twain said, "When I was 15, I thought my old man was the dumbest guy around. By the time I turned 21, I was sur-prised at how much the old man had learned in six years." Indeed.

Watching my daughter play organized soccer or run through a gym-nastics routine and playing catch with my son offer an opportunity to reflect on the coaches I had as a boy, the people who had a profound effect on my career and ultimately, the way my life is playing out.

Of course, there were many. Heck we all have. Most good, some indif-ferent, a few bad, but always a handful who come back to you time and again. And always when you are in a position of authority, needing guidance to provide the right combination of instruction, discipline, caring and an undefinable, enigmatic charisma that somehow separates you from other teachers, coaches and parents, and transforms the voice of authority from man to myth.

Like many boys, the fortunate anyway, my foremost teacher, coach or counselor and hero-supreme was my Dad. I knew it when I was ten, and I knew it when I was 20, but again, you never fully appreciate a person until they are gone, and you must walk a mile in their shoes. I still learn from this man's examples, 20 odd years after he checked out.

My first running coach was a pseudo rogue named Leon Santa Cruz. As an alternate on the US Olympic Team in 1960, he had the experi-ence, but more importantly, he had the intangible ability to mold young athletes in a manner that allowed them to discover for themselves what made us tick. As a 14 year old high school cross country runner, Coach Santa Cruz helped me build a foundation of discipline and commitment, but more importantly, a pure and untainted love of running that still burns inside today.

Even earlier, as an eleven year old third baseman for the Valley View Auto Parts Red Sox, Coach Dave Stith, who I still think about from time to time, took a smart aleck preteen and made it evident by example that in this day and age, there are very few things as constructive and rewarding as a simple game of ball with your buddies in the park. And simple though it may have been, the intrinsic lessons that filter down from coach to player, from father to son, and generation to generation are not found in any book.

I have not had many coaches in my adult life. And excluding the Master's swim coaches on the pool deck, my entire athletic career I have been self-coached, choosing the experiental tract over the empirical, lingering possibly to long in "lifestyle" made, rather than following a rapidly developing support group. But while this method may have cost me a few "career performances," I do not think I would have lasted 18 years under an East German routine—or at least it wouldn't have been as enjoyable.

Looking around, there his a tremendous opportunity to access information about training, about equipment, about events, and if you look in the right places, about life. Count them up. Videos to show you a perfect swim stroke, books by the dozen explaining everything from asthma for athletes to Zen and the art of time-trialing. Computer services to find training partners and used derailleurs for sale; clinics and camps to vacation and network at (and maybe learn something). And yes, personalized triathlon coaching is alive and prospering.

All of these are positive, if not exciting developments of our sports.

It would be safe to say that most triathletes don't have ten years like Scott Molina and I did to experiment with various types of programs, running down tips, ideas, concepts and a few empty trails along the way in search of the right combination of mileage, intensity and number of Bud Lights consumed.

No, it's better this way. Just strap on the heart monitor, pull up the day's workout on the screen, bang it out, download the data, fax it to the coach, the nutritionist and the physiologist, and wait for their reply on your cellular phone as you have your blood lactate analyzed.

Or is it?

WHY TRI? A PHILOSOPHY OF ENDURANCE

Why? Not how or when or where, but why? The ubiquitous question surrounding any discussion of endurance feats or the philosophy of great personal challenges is always why. And while it's easy to expand the mystique and foster legends by taking the "because it's there" approach, I think that's more of a cop-out than a comprehensive look at why people attempt activities that are viewed by mere mortals as either godly or insane. There is a season for everything, right?

Each feat of endurance has its own reasoning behind it. The motivations and rationale are as varied as the individuals themselves. There may be a common thread somewhere, but we can only theorize about what it is.

Endurance ability may be a state of mind, it may be a personality trait or it may just be a way to stand out in an increasingly crowded world– a vehicle in which to swim against the stream.

Endurance feats are, if nothing else, relative to the participant. One more mile, one more mountain, one more time around the block; one man's marathon is another man's seven-inning softball game. The common denominator is to go one step, if not many, beyond what is "comfortable bearable." The further one goes, the harder one pushes, and the greater the rewards that lie out there in some zone of accomplishment.

Human attempts to reach this zone have evolved over the years and sometimes appear overly commercial and even recreational. Adventurer extraordinaire Will Steiger recently completed a trek across Antarctica in which he spent an estimated $11 million in investors' and sponsors' dollars. This highly publicized trip was in complete contrast to a concurrent trans-antarctic trek by the famous mountain climber Reinhold Messner from Südtirol. Messner's team completed its excursion for under $1 million and said very little to the press about it. This doesn't mean that one trip was more personally rewarding than the other. What it does say is that in this day and age, people will go to great lengths to produce an endurance experience, for personal or financial rewards.

Looking back 100 years, people didn't ride their bikes 80 miles for fun. Life, especially outside the larger cities, was hard enough. For those who settled the West, every day was an endurance event. Growing or hunting food, surviving freezing winters and avoiding deadly disease were 19th century triathlons. As the country grew and technology developed, comforts increased and life indeed became easier–at least physically. In a largely agricultural society, where men and women worked long, hard hours raising crops or livestock, you didn't have to go to an aerobics class to get a little exercise. (But in urban life today, you don't have the personal satisfaction that comes with hunting for your dinner or building a roof for your family's home.)

So we create our own challenges, our own formidable tasks. Recreational though they may be (the consequences of not finishing a six-mile run are a little less severe than failing to store enough food for the winter), they are still personal mountains we all choose to climb or not. In that sense, participant oriented endurance events are truly unique to the last 40 years. Before that, world wars and the Depression limited such frivolous activities.

Yet the preparation and execution of a "frivolous" endurance sporting event can completely consume lives. How many of us have known someone who nearly lost a job or spouse as they honed in on their first marathon or triathlon? The buildup is part of the process. The longer, harder and more thoroughly one prepares, the greater the chance of not only reaching the goals, but of attaining whatever intrinsic rewards there are to be had at the 20th mile, or the 50th lap. Moreover, if you think about it, when you're standing on the starting line, or at the base of the mountain, as ready as you can be, you're already ahead of the pack. In a race against the over-spectated couch potatoes that constitute the majority in this country, you've won before the gun is fired.

Competition is not always a necessary element in the endurance equation. It is just another factor in the challenge process. Many rugged individuals have set out on personal treks with no one, but their shadow for company. These are the people who sail around the world solo, ski Mount Everest and circumnavigate the globe in an experimental plane. They even include the neighbor who swears he's going to run a 10K someday. The guy next-door may actually share traits with the guy who races his motorcycle over 1,000 miles of Mexican desert. He may discover the same things about himself at the fifth mile of his 10K that a sailor does when he finds himself becalmed in the South Pacific.

Self-knowledge appears to be a player in this game, but its' one of those things that you don't really talk about. It blows the whole experience when you go on Johnny Carson and tell the world how you found yourself while on a cross-country bike ride. A deep, personal experience should remain just that–personal and deep. Ask Reinhold Messner.

UNFORGETTABLE...

I was talking to a friend on the phone last Sunday night. It was after 9:00 p.m. and he told me he had to hang up so that he could go out for a quick four-mile run. Figuring it was a joke, I pushed the question, "Are you nuts? It's cold, dark and late. What have you been doing all day?" He replied, "I just went through my training log for this week and I came up four miles short of my requisite minimum mileage." "Hey," I replied, "I ran 18 this morning in the rain and you're crazier than I am."

His answer was, "My log is all I have to show for these endless miles."

I felt slightly sorry for this guy who is a bit of a slave to the pen and pad, but to a certain extent he has a point. I've never really kept a log for any length of time, and the thousands of miles I've endured and enjoyed over the years have more or less fused together into a bittersweet memory of sweat and smiles. I don't really regret not documenting my workouts like some folks do, I'm just not that cerebral. Yet there are times I wish I had a more concrete history of my exploits on the roads and waters of Southern California.

A few workouts however, I'll always remember. These were brutal torture sessions that had a unique twist about them–something that made them indelible in my "most outrageous" file. There was this one bike ride–a fairly typical Wednesday ride a few years back. Seventy-plus riders started, and Scott Molina, tiring of the squirreling riders in the pack, suggested that a few of us head East, away from the crowd. Four or five of us turned off the coast, looking forward to a somewhat mellow 60-mile loop. When we looked behind, some 25 "bikies" had followed, thinking we knew a short cut or something. Molina groaned, looked at the group, noticed the very small freewheels most of them had for the relatively flat coastal ride, and made one quick decision–to head for the hills. He knew of a series of climbs tucked away in the back country that would make a grown gear-head cry.

It was hilarious watching a dozen cyclists zig-zag their way up these beast-like grades while Molina and a few lucky "tri-geeks" cruised up with their 23-tooth sprockets. About four hours into the ride we were still a long way from home. During a quick food stop, Molina bought and consumed a six pack of Coke. I knew the next hour wasn't going to be fun, but all I had to do was hang on until his inevitable blood-sugar crash.

The ride lasted way over 100 miles and left a trail of stragglers that wouldn't be coming in until dark. We still talk about that ride–especially the look on the faces of the cyclists when they figured out that it wasn't the usual Wednesday route.

Another workout that stands out happened eight days before the 1987 Bud Light Ironman. Kenny Souza and I decided to go to the local high school track and run four or five 440s to test our leg speed before leaving for Kona the next day.

It was late afternoon and very cloudy in San Diego. We ran four pretty hard, trying to outdo the other, and I remember thinking I shouldn't do anymore of these. Kenny suggested two more easy. Right. He had to be just a step ahead of me. Kenny is pretty fast on the track so I figured I'd suggest a couple more and burn him out. No way.

We ended up running ten quarters with a 110-yard jog between each. After getting trounced on the final one, it started to rain. I suggested a warm down. Of course I smoked the warm down just to keep the youngster in his place.

From then on it was war. Twelve, 14, 16, 18 440s without a word. It was getting dark now and the track was a muddy mess. About number 15, a broker stopped by the track with some papers for me to sign. He looked at me soaked in sweat, mud and rain, sunglasses still in place. While I signed the papers he said, "You earn your money, S.T." That got me psyched.

Back to the track. I lost count after 25, but it had become a duel with Souza and I wasn't going to lose. I don't know how many 440s we ran that night-, but I remember getting home around nine PM and thinking that I wouldn't forget that workout for a long time. Unfortunately, my legs wouldn't forget either. They were flat for weeks.

The only other workout I distinctly remember is a three-mile ocean swim I did with a group of people from the University of California, San Diego Masters Swim Team. We swam a large, triangle course across a bay that places you a long way from shore at certain points. We were about halfway through and I was glad to be with the lead pack when something grabbed my foot. I turned around and it was some swim head who had snuck around the pack and came up from behind. He laughed as he swam off after the pack. I wasn't so amused as I tried in vain to catch the group, only to watch them swim away, leaving me to swim a mile and a half by myself, out where the "men in gray suits" hang out. That was one workout I haven't forgotten.

MY LIFE IN THE 80S

One of the best parts about New Year's Eve is watching one of those special "Year in Review" shows that encapsulates all the memorable events that transpired over the past year. Each event usually triggers a thought that places you in a certain time and place that corresponds to what happened–kind of like a rapid-fire nostalgic history review.

Within the decade closing down, I expected a whole slew of "Life in the 80s" specials. And along with it, a chance to briefly reflect on just what the hell I did over the past ten years. Not that I could change history, but something about "destined to repeat it" kept flashing in my subconscious.

Well, for a variety of reasons, it never happened. The papers had their token recap of the year's major tragedies. There were a few decent magazine articles, and television, well, I gave up on the tube in 1982 when the last episode of M.A.S.H. was aired. But it just wasn't there. No final and complete version of all the notable newsworthy clips of the past ten years. So I did my own.

While most of the things that I remember that meant anything are either completely irrelevant to "Joe Triathlon" or not for public consumption, there are a few that carry some weight and should be duly noted for posterity's sake.

• Nice, France, October 1983, 2:30 a.m. I am rooming with Gary Peterson and neither of us can sleep. He turns on the light and starts reading a six-year-old Playboy. I say something about wishing I had pancakes and try to get back to sleep. The next thing I hear is Gary pouring batter into a hot frying pan that he has brought in his bike box. We spend the next two hours eating pancakes with maple syrup, reading his ancient Playboy and getting ready to sleep all day.

• I remember competing in the 1983 Horny Toad Triathlon (a once prestigious event) and having to swim the 1.5-mile course straight out and straight back. Have you ever been three quarters of a mile from shore? It was some lifeguard's idea of a joke. Real funny.

• In 1984 I crossed the finish line of a very disorganized race in Sydney, Australia. With no one in sight behind me, I thought I had won easily until I saw my nearest competitor sprinting toward the finish line from the opposite direction. Fortunately, I crossed first and somehow avoided the near head-on collision. Now how did that happen?

• The first real massage I ever received was the night before the October 1982 Ironman by a huge Hawaiian lady. She released toxins that had been in my body for 25 years. The next morning, I could barely get out of bed. Smart thinking, S.T.

• In the ill-fated Bahamas Triathlon of the Stars in 1983, Tom Warren broke his front wheel, and then got a lift back to the exact spot where he broke down, before continuing on in the event. Think about it. Would you do that?

• In 1986 I went to Sweden and stayed with my wife and Scott Molina before the Säter Triathlon. Scott tried to switch time zones for the first couple of days and then gave up. Since it never got dark that far north in the summer, he would just train all night long, come home at six in the morning and sleep all day. After dinner at night, he'd wake up and head off on a bike ride.

• At the 1989 Ironman, I took off my swimsuit before the bike ride, forgetting that my running shorts were cut very short, split at the sides and had no brief inside. End of story.

• In the spring of 1989, Virginia, Torrie and I traveled from the St. Croix race directly to the World Cup in Australia–virtually halfway around the world. When we got there, the race organizers picked us up at the airport, took care of all the baggage and generally treated us like kings. We were whisked to a five-star hotel and a great meal. The hospitality and the overall professionalism of the event made the trip well worthwhile. Mark that race on your calendar.

• In 1989, at that start of the Tugs Tavern Swim-Run-Swim, the starter fired the gun, threw it to an official and sprinted down the beach to catch the pack. I thought to myself, who is this guy?

• During the swim of the Tooheys Great Lakes Ironman Triathlon in 1984 (pre-wetsuit days) I nearly froze from hypothermia. At one point, about a mile into the course, I stopped and asked a lifeguard on a surf-board if I could borrow his wetsuit. In 59-degree water, and cold, over-cast skies, he says, "No worries, mate," takes it off and throws it to me while I'm treading water. There was no way I could get in it. To this day, though, I don't think I've met an Aussie I didn't like.

• During the start of one of the first Ironman events in Kona, a disgrun-tled fisherman drove his boat right into the swim start as a sort of pro-test. He was later arrested by the Coast Guard. I remember seeing the prop turning under water about five feet from my head. Outrageous!

• In 1983, Team J. David rented a bunch of houses [for their team members competing in the Ironman] near the Mauna Kea Hotel, right on the golf course for over $500 a night, each. For one week I was the only one in a 4,000-square foot custom-home. Decadence at its finest!

IRONMAN REDUX

"If dreams were thunder, and lightening was desire, this old house
would have burned down a long time ago."
Angel from Montgomery, John Prine

Some people divide their year up on a calendar, looking at each January 1 as the start of something new. Some people use the seasons, beginning with spring and new growth. Others have a fiscal year whereby the books begin and end, usually along with profits and losses, both real and imagined. But for a serious athlete, the year seems to begin with pre-season training and always end with "the big event." Each sport has its year-end spectacle–a tournament, a series, a playoff, however it's labeled. It's a time and place for all the athletes to dump their eggs and local merchants to hawk cheesy T-shirts, but above all else it's a way to mark another year, a cusp of old and new. And there always seem to be some ripping parties afterward.

In triathlon, that event is the Hawaiian Ironman. It's always been "the big one" and probably always will be. Ironman has withstood a barrage of tactical assaults over the years, but still retains the numero uno slot. The folks standing on the corner in Trenton, New Jersey, have never heard of the ITU, but they have seen Ironman somewhere.

The aura of Ironman makes people do strange things just to earn a start number. Organizers have been offered up to 10,000 bucks (in small, unmarked bills) just for a chance to torture themselves for a day on a barren stretch of lava-ringed road; that certainly says something about our little subculture of endurance athletes, doesn't it? Nevertheless, Ironman time is nearly here again and I'm flashing not only on how some 1400-odd people will each approach it, but how I will look upon the event, feel it, prepare for it, internalize it, and ultimately swallow "the big one"–one more time.

Anything done in repetition changes; it is a learning process, a method to mastery. But as familiarity induces skill, it also breeds contempt. Sometimes I think that my best Ironman races are behind me, not because of my age, but simply because of the fact that I have raced in close to 40 of the damned things. I know what it takes to win.

As great as the layman may believe the sacrifice to be, he cannot fully comprehend what is involved unless he or she essentially puts his or her life on hold for three to four months so that all possible energy systems can focus on one Saturday in October. Just to have the means, the opportunity to do this once in your life is both a blessing and a curse. In all my years of triathlon, I have known of only one person who did it right once and then walked away. His name is Mike Plant.

For me, October 15 will be blessing/curse number 15, I think. I will approach it differently than other years, of course, hopefully building on experience, without allowing repetition and sameness to drag me down like a tired and cynical old politician. I suppose one must take kindly the council of years, grasp what feverish energy youth and the event itself can exude in the end–follow blind ambition. Just like I did in Ironman No. 1

But it isn't No. 1 and no matter how much the event or the participants or I try to make it new and fresh and innocent, we cannot. We can only accept Ironman, the sport it mirrors and our own personal relationship with it as it is.

I cannot train for this race the way I did in 1981 or 1985 or 1991 because my life is different than it was during those years. And for the most part, neither can any repeat competitor. But we can adapt, customize and mold this year's event around our present lives and add another mark, another memory and maybe another medal to the shelf.

Hardware or no hardware, this is not the beginning and it is certainly is not the end. Ironman is an ongoing process, a lifestyle if you will, another page in the photo album.

IRONMAN LEGENDS AND LORE

Every year, thousands of people from dozen of countries around the world vie for a starting slot in the Hawaiian Ironman. There are many other triathlons that challenge Hawaii for overall organization. Most any other event is easier. And heaven knows, there are more scenic courses. Yet David Yates, president of World Triathlon Corporation, owners of the Ironman event, has been offered everything from Caribbean vacations to $10,000 in cash for one of the 1,400 starting spots.

What generates so much interest, so much demand for punishing yourself for a day? Well, that's easy. It's the history of the event, the mystery and the mystique. Even if other triathlons have their own versions of personal heroism and intrigue, none has provided so many for so long with so much media exposure to tell the world these tales... as the Hawaii Ironman.

It is the seemingly inconsequential yet personal acts of valor, chronicled in the newspaper and in the magazines, that spark the interest of the athletes's "everyman;" the obligatory "day-in-the-life" segment detailed on the television coverage that sends a message to triathletes everywhere, initiating the little voice inside that says, "I want–no I *need* to do that event!"

Maybe some of the tales are blown out of proportion, the authors and editors taking poetic license with the story. For example, there was this little piece on one of the television segments about a competitor who was diagnosed with cancer, but went on to race anyway, because she just had to do it before she died. Well, to make a long story short, she didn't really have cancer, and somebody, somewhere, had mud on his face. But, heck, it made for great TV!

One of my favorites is the story of a young, inexperienced competitor in the 1979 Ironman which was held on the island of Oahu. During the final portions of a particularly long day (and night), he hailed a pass-

17

ing paper boy during the early morning hours for a paper, to check the results of the event he was still competing in.

Also notable is the reply made by an ABC-TV camera crew when it was suggested that it had possibly aided John Howard, in his incredible bike ride en route to his 1981 victory, by driving their van in front of him for a large segment of the bike course. That was not the case, the crew replied, "because the front windows and rear doors were open, allowing the wind to come through."

Few people recall the time a pig carcass was tied to the turnaround buoy by a disgruntled local fisherman or when an equally unhappy boat captain drove his 35-foot fishing boat right into the start of the swim, later to be arrested by local authorities.

How about the pre-1982 races when competitors had to stop two or three times during the race to be weighed, assuring medical officials that they were not in a serious state of hydration? I know a couple of guys who weren't taking any chances, stepping onto the scales with half a dozen rolls of quarters in their jersey pockets.

While I seem to recall the more bizarre and unusual incidents, every athlete who has raced on the stretch of lava known as the Kona Coast has his or her own memories of the event that composed their day under the hot Hawaiian sun. And while media will always continue to seek out the events that make for "good copy," the competitors themselves will continue to write their own stories; creating personal legends to either pass on to their kids or better yet, hold inside themselves to be brought out like an old photo scrapbook, when something inside, without reason or warning, compels them to stop everything and take a little ride through one October Saturday past.

THE DIARY OF SCOTT TINLEY–STILL CRAZY AFTER ALL THESE YEARS

One of my high school teachers used to say, "The only dumb question is the one that never gets asked." I try to remember that every time I do a clinic or get cornered at an expo by some guy who has "just one more quick question." Honestly, I don't mind. I do the same thing when I put myself in an environment which I very much want to know more about.

But the one question that used to get to me was when someone asked, "What do you think about when you are training?" Come on, I say to myself, How should I know? "I try to focus on technique and keeping my effort where it should be." It is a valid question that should command an honest answer. So I thought about it and started to answer as straightforwardly as I could.

"I think about the same things while I am training as I do when I'm not training," became my honest, but somewhat cynical-sounding reply. I could usually follow that up with something like, "And if anybody else who trains as much as I do tells you he concentrates on technique and effort 50 hours a week, they're either a liar or brain-dead." That usually pisses them off or busts them up.

In reality, though, there are ways to keep your mind on the training without burning yourself out. Over the last 15 years, by accident or experiment, I've tried quite a few diversionary tactics.

To give you an example of the methods that have prevented my madness, I've selected a few excerpts from my log book. Upon reviewing my list, a pattern with dangerous implications became apparent. If I last another five years in this sport, it could get weird. Check it out...

December 12, 1977, a.m. Have been at this sport for over a year now and decided to do my first 100-mile bike ride. A friend of mine was driving to L.A. from San Diego, so I decided to hitch a ride up and bicycle back. The odometer in the car said 106 miles from door to drop-off point. Figured I'd take two candy bars for energy and $5 for lunch. If I average 25 m.p.h. (which I did easily when I rode the 10-mile Bike for Breath Ride last week) and stop at least once for 15 minutes to eat, I should be home at least 30 minutes before dark. No problem.

December 12, 1977, p.m. Forgot I couldn't ride on the freeway. Surface streets must have added another 30-plus miles. Ride took me nine hours, 16 minutes–the last four hours in the dark. Ran out of food, money, spare tubes, and courage. I learned though: Always bring your Walkman.

June 1, 1979. Ran with my friend Bob this morning. He called early and said he was going for a long slow one and be sure to bring along a few bucks for breakfast (which I thought we'd get after the run). Anyway, I asked him where we were headed, and all he said was "North." So we left his house and headed north on the Pacific Coast Highway for roughly one hour. We stopped near a 7-Eleven and he pulled a $20 bill from his sock and proceeded to buy a half-gallon of Coke and three cupcakes while I ran around in circles in the parking lot.

After Bob finished his "breakfast" I headed back in the direction of his house. No, he told me, we haven't reached the turnaround yet. Long story short–we ended up running 30 some miles, stopped four times for food and gained two pounds for the effort.

April 9, 1982. Decided I'd look for a new route through the hills today. I look on a map and see that if I follow one small squiggly line it will eventually come back to a main road that I know well.

After two hours on the small road, it turns into dirt. No problem. I need to clean my bike anyway. Another hour on this dirt road and I'm a little concerned, until I see a shack of a house just ahead.

Suddenly, this guy right out of the movie "Deliverance" comes out of the front door wearing blue-jean overalls and carrying a shot gun. I say, "Good afternoon, sir. I'm lost." He replies, "Turn your little faggot bicycle right around and get the hell off my property." I was out of there so fast you wouldn't believe it. It's funny now, but not at the time.

November 14, 1984. Decided to swim with Tom Warren this morning. All of the best pools are closed, but Tom says he has the key to the Plunge (a 30-year-old indoor 50-yard relic that was slated for major renovation). We have to go through the old boiler room to get in, and the place is deserted on this Sunday morning. Tom decides he is going to do 50 x 100 yards on the 1:30. Fun, I go along for the first 40 and decide I've had enough.

As I'm walking through the darkened empty hallways toward the shower, I see another figure near the corner. This guy yells at me and threatens to call the police for breaking and entering. It turns out to be the pool supervisor, who normally is off on Sundays and was unaware that Tom had been using the pool.

August 14, 1987. Wanted to do a two-hour ride today, but also needed to pick a few things up at the store, including some red/brown stain for the backyard fence. After deciding to run errands on my bike, I brought along a chain lock so that I could lock my bike while I went into the paint store. On my way home, I hit a patch of oil on the road and crashed my bike. The red/brown can of stain opened up in my jersey pocket and ran all down my back and legs. Since I was only a few miles from home, I decided just to ride home and get cleaned up.

You should have seen the look on my neighbor's face when I pulled into the drive with a chain around my waist, a huge blood-red stain all over my legs and dirt and asphalt on my arms. I said, "Triathlons are no picnic, pal," and went into the house laughing to myself.

THE TRAVELIN' MAN–EXPAND YOUR MIND BY RACING IN NEW PLACES

When I graduated from high school, I had two choices regarding what to do next: get a job and pay my way through college or pay my way through college by getting a job. I had a friend who faced a dilemma most unlike mine. His parents, who had socked away more than enough money for his higher education, posed this choice: "With this money, you can either put yourself through school or we can send you on a six-month trip around the world. It's your decision."

I didn't understand it at the time, but this guy's parents were offering two entirely different ways to learn about life. No doubt they understood that, while books and teachers are important in the learning process, ultimately, the world as a classroom has no peer.

Go Global

In recent years, triathlon has become a truly international sport. Dozens of countries now stage events and field top-notch competitors. Our sport evolves as other peoples and cultures take up triathlon, contributing variations and flavors not quite envisioned years ago by those crazies in Mission Bay.

In France, for example, it's a common occurrence for dozens of cyclist to escort the lead runner to the finish line. In Japan, the aid stations aren't complete without seaweed and coffee.

The opportunity to travel the world and experience many cultures and nations, under the guise of being a pro triathlete, has been a priceless gift. I've seen and done things I would never have had the chance to experience otherwise. Yet one doesn't have to travel the ends of the earth to taste the freedom of a traveling sportsman. It's as easy as hitching your bicycle to the roof of your car and heading into the next zip code to race the local boys.

There's a certain joy in the simple process of travel, and when you add the pursuit of a passion, such as racing, watch out: It might become a lifestyle.

One of my first road trips was to the Santa Barbara Triathlon in 1980. I went by myself, and since I couldn't afford a hotel I slept on the beach in a sleeping bag. When I awoke, I was tired and disoriented and then alarmed by the scantily clad people with orange heads walking around my bedroom. Once I figured out who and where I was, I thought how fortunate I was to be able to walk 20 meters to the starting line.

A Sense of Discovery

Traveling leads to a sense of discovery not easily found when sticking about the old homestead. Because you're not at home, you feel more alive; your senses are on alert. I did a triathlon in Guam once, and it was the only time I ever saw a shark in the water during the swim. Strangely, I wasn't scared. I figured that this was his home and I was the one doing the trespassing.

That's the kind of experience that sticks with you, a memory that adds spice to what often becomes just another summer. Traveling can be uncomfortable, even frightening, but that's all part of the trip.

Once I returned from South America with a wad of cash (the prize money was paid in $100 bills) and spent the better part of the day explaining to custom officials just what a triathlon is.

Appreciate the Bizarre

Traveling to events, you have to expect–and try to welcome–the bizarre and unexpected. Just think of any strange episode as another entry into your scrapbook to be savored at another time. For me, the best discoveries are in people themselves. When you think about it, we are all so different, it's amazing we can communicate. Yet, for the most part, we get by and get along.

I had the laugh the other day when Ray Browning told me about an

African runner with whom he had been in a photography session. When Ray asked the runner how old he was, the shrugged and said, "I do not know. My mother has said that I came during the year of the big spring rain."

This was enough for him, and it is certainly enough for us.

ON THE ROAD AGAIN

So, I'm thinking maybe it's time for a brief change of venue, a change of M.O. Just a few days out of my element to see how the other side lives, the way it used to be and soon will be again.

Without a clear medium to accomplish the goal of increasing my appreciation of how good things really are, I gravitate toward the ultimate solution to every problem: the road trip. And as every post-nuclear, pseudo-child of the 60s knows, the secret to a really meaningful road trip is to depart unprepared yet resolved.

Fellow Tri-human Todd Jacobs and I would provision the Tinley box van with only the essentials (one mountain bike, two guitars, a case of PowerBars, some Endura, a half-dozen hats and MY credit card) and drive 500 miles to the Cactus Cup mountain bike race. All we knew was that it was in Phoenix the following day. Any additional info would only clutter the agenda and detract from the task at hand. Whatever that was.

You see, I've always felt that the trappings of success can begin to taint a person's peace of mind and upset the delicate balance between appreciation and lust.

In other words, when you begin to acquire a lot of shit, you lose your feel for the little things. And when people tell someone they're bitchin' enough times, they start to believe it—even if they're not.

So we motor through the desert at warp speed, alternating blues with folk CDs, and cruise into Phoenix no worse for wear, excluding a small piece of paper that reads "87 in a 55 m.p.h. zone." No worries here, though. A signed poster for that judge will make things right.

Checking into the hotel, we discover that we will not be checking into the hotel. Even the "I can't believe you don't have my reservation" bit doesn't work. There is definitely no room at this inn. No worries here, either.

We simply set up camp in the parking lot behind the Seventh Day Adventist Church. (This locale was chosen for the later times of Sunday service the following morning, plus the proximity of a donut shop with a "free coffee" sign in the window.) Besides, sometimes you just feel more at home in the back of a van than a fancy hotel.

Finding the race site would be easy. Just follow the steady stream of cars with bikes on their roofs heading out of town in the pre-dawn hours.

Locating a place to park among the 2,000 entrants is another story. It's amazing how close you get to the starting line with a well-placed $20 bill, though. Hey, parking attendants have to earn a living, too.

OK, now all we need to do is sign up (no freebies here as we get fully retailed, including a 1994 NORBA license) and track down the dude who as supposed to build up my new Yeti.

When I finally find my ride, the frame looks great, the fork looks great, the wheels look great, and trick TNT parts look great. Unfortunately, all of the above are still separated from one another. No worries; I've got 20 minutes until my race; and I can scrounge a rig somewhere. Warming up takes half the fun out of the first climb, anyway. A fourth cup of coffee does the same thing.

Billy J. from Oakley loans me his coolest Yeti Arc, my size and everything. I promptly lie with a straight face, "I'll take good care of it, bro."

Lesson #12 of the weekend: Age-groupers are just as serious as the pros. Cool, I think. I'll dice it up for a piece of hardware. But the big difference between mountain bikers and tri-heads is... oh, never mind.

After the race, I ride another lap because the course is so fun. And, I'm not so sure the officials dig this, but I need the time to come up with an explanation for the condition of Billy's bike.

Looking at the results, I either (a) won my division by two minutes; (b) was DQed for not declaring I was a professional in a similar sport and competing in the appropriate category; or (c) was thrown out for the aforementioned "extra lap." No worries. All of those would be agreeable to me. I was just too stoked to argue.

Back in the van. Hendrix blasting. A stop at the Scottsdale Charthouse for an assault on the "pinch me, I'm in Heaven" salad bar and a quick 500-mile jam back to San Diego. When I get home, I'm toast.

Walking in the front door, the family doesn't even get off the couch, let alone smother me with welcome home kisses. A bit later, it's, "You spent two days away from home and didn't earn a penny?"

It's OK, though. I've got the bug again. "Hey, can anybody give me a lift to the nationals?"

PROSE FROM A PRO

Not many years ago, one of the modern-day self-helpist borrowed from the ancient saying, "We are what we think about," and created his own career-tract axiom, "We become what we are." Loosely translated, the entrepreneur was saying that many of us ultimately end up in careers that, more likely than not, are made up of people just like us.

I agree with that theory. It may take a few tries, but the opportunities being what they are in the late 20th century, most individuals will land themselves in a field that they feel comfortable, if not compatible, with.

I say this because sometimes I think about why and how I landed in the profession that I did. One of the reasons that continues to surface is that, often the perception (and many times the reality), is that there is substantially less politics, less favoritism and less general bullshit in the field of professional athletics than, say, in a large manufacturing company.

I suppose that many of us with the God-given talent, luck, means and tenacity that earn a living in running shoes were and are attracted to sports because we believed we would succeed and fail on our own accord without political influence or the need for a quintessential brown nose. For the most part, I believe this to be true.

Sports for money, though, is never a completely altruistic endeavor. Neither is amateur sports, for that matter. From the Little League coach playing his son more than the others to International Olympic Committee members rewarding favored nations with program inclusions, athletics are not immune from subjectivity and personal agenda. People always have looked out, and always will, for number one.

You don't have to look very far and very deep into professional sports to uncover enough treachery, collusion and manipulation to make one sick. Where we might suspect a certain amount of inequity in corporate life, the viewing public doesn't see it in sports because they don't want to see it; don't want to know about it.

That's okay, though. It would be overly fatalistic to focus on the hidden acts of miscreancy. Too much is to be gained from the countless acts of personal valor and cooperative spirit played out of the grassy fields of the world.

But every sport needs a watchdog. An unbiased individual or group without personal agendas and dreams of power and money who doesn't necessarily police, but simply asks hard questions of others who appear to cross the line and play their sons too long because they're the coach. Yes, the sport of triathlon could use a watchdog right now.

When I elected to become a professional sportsman, in other words, to earn money by competing, I knew very little of the business side of sport. My motivations were primal–feed and house my wife and I with prize money. But any elite athlete knows that in order to reach your potential, you must divorce yourself from the crass dealings of commerce and focus on the task at hand–covering ground faster than the next guy.

Great performances are usually attained when motivated by deep personal longings for success and a hot burning desire to achieve one's maximum capacity–not because the athlete has a big sponsor bonus on the line.

Above all else, any athlete, whether professional or weekend warrior, must know and answer to themselves alone. You can't wax mystical, telling the press you compete for cryptic religious reasons and then scratch because appearance money is too low. And you can't let the backroom political maneuvering prevent you from finding whatever small personal Holy Grail that each of us seeks on the trails and at the finish line.

The race had been very painful, very hard. I had held on to the tail end of the lead group through a blistering swim and bike, knowing that visual contact was my last hope to stay "in the hunt." Getting off the bike, no fewer than seven guys bolted out of the transition area like it was on fire and their tails were catching. I put my second shoe on, looked up and found myself in another zip code than the leaders. Oh, well.

Running the first seven miles was not too terribly uncomfortable. Having learned to turn the pain on and off like a hot water valve, I was luke warm at best today. But, I thought I might test the pipes "just for the hell of it."

For me, it is times like that which make it all worth it. All the trials, all the miles, all the emotional investment. Not that I was going to win: far from it. I was hoping only for a top-five slot. But it's something to be able to say to yourself, "Okay, you're not feeling that bad. Let's see what you got here; just turn this dial up a few notches and see what comes out." It's something to feel the heat, the lungs and the mind begin to work in harmony, like a well-oiled machine that happily adjusts to a higher RPM, and to feel the basic child-like thrill of speed come back to you like a prodigal son.

It's times like this also when I feel like Walter Mitty, living out a fantasy that millions of child athletes dream about. No one ever said it was going to be easy, and I suppose I would have been naive to think it would always be fair. But in the grander scheme of things, we athletes of all shapes and sizes have it pretty damn good.

We can find such heroism as there is without going to war or saving a life. All we have to do is get up before the sun and head out the door to be alone with the road and our thoughts. And in a crowded and confusing world, that is something indeed.

ST and a Decade of Triathlon

Ten years of *Triathlete Magazine*. Wow! On the advice of the magazine editors, I have endeavored to pen some poignant and poetic reflections of my involvement with this illustrious publication over the past decade. This would surely be a fitting opportunity to spin a tale or two of *Triathlete's* contribution to our sport (and maybe expose or embarrass some of its staff in the process). But all I can think of is Jerry Garcia's line from The Grateful Dead song, "Truckin"–"What a long strange trip it's been."

I did, however, develop a few ponderous top tens for your consumption, and digestion, if you can swallow them.

The ten strangest things I've ever seen while racing
1. During the 1983 Ironman, a van drove past me and my brother, with a guy hanging out the side door taking pictures. A quarter-mile later, he fell out at 30 miles per hour and rolled to a stop only a few feet from us.

2. Topless bathing is not uncommon in the south of France, but it is usually confined to the beach. However, on a rare occasion, one of the ladies will stand up and walk over to cheer the runners as they pass by during the Nice Triathlon. If you are not expecting it, it will take you aback.

3. Warming up in the pre-dawn hours prior to one of the early St. Croix races, I saw two guys in a knife fight in an alley not far from the start.

4. Racing in France in the mid-80s, I caught a cyclist whose seat had fallen off of its rails, forcing him to ride standing up. A mile later he passed me back with a makeshift water-bottle seat.

5. I had to stop for a herd of sheep one time in New Zealand. Two hun-

dred of those chops weren't about to move quickly, either.

6. During the televised "Survival of the Fittest" contest, one of the "downhill running" races was halted mid-race and restarted because the cameraman had failed to get a good shot of the start.

7. In the 1981 Ironman, I came upon a couple of cyclists in the race who had the map of the course on their handlebar packs. How do you get lost in Hawaii?

8. While running on a golf course during one of the Bud Light USTS Florida races, I watched a 5-foot alligator getting out of one of the man-made lakes.

9. Atlanta Bud Light USTS 1984: I'm out of the water over a minute back, but catch the leaders early on the bike because they all had to wait for a park ranger to open a gate that was blocking the bike course.

10. In the ill-fated event called "The Diamond Triathlon of the Stars" in San Francisco, circa 1984, the race director failed to tell the participants that his permits had been canceled the night before the race. So, about 200 athletes kind of "staged" a race the best they could and then went on search-and-destroy mission for the promoter who failed to make the start and was headed out of town posthaste.

The ten hardest things to do in triathlon
1. Go to a triathlon just to watch.
2. Get your picture on the cover of *Triathlete*.
3. Explain your hairless legs to fellow office workers.
4. Paying the airlines to take your bike on the plane.
5. Resist the temptation to have a third plate of spaghetti at the carbo dinner.
6. Resist using a hotel towel to clean your bike.
7. Remember that your bikes are still on the roof rack when you pull into the garage.
8. Finding room in your drawer for another race finisher's T-shirt.

9. Explaining to your 5-year-old why Mark Allen won the race and you didn't.

10. Walking down stairs the morning after an Ironman.

Ten things we would all like to see happen in the next ten years

1. Cat Sports pay the Coke Grand Prix prize money they owe the athletes from 1992 Bud Light Triathlon Series.

2. More Pro-Am, women-only and kid's triathlons.

3. Tri-Fed rules and regulations based on safety and fairness, not politics.

4. More winter, mountain bike and off-road triathlons.

5. Scott Molina and Dave Scott to come out of retirement.

6. An electronic draft-busting system attached to every competitor's bike.

7. An energy tax rebate for people who ride their bike more that they drive their car.

8. A multi-day stage race triathlon and a lucrative masters circuit. (OK, so that's on my wish list; it's my column).

9. More porta-johns at race starts.

10. A walnut/raisin/Kahlua-flavored PowerBar.

Chapter 2

Who Are These Guys?

Dragons live forever, but not so little boys,
Painted wings and giant rings make way for other toys.
"Puff the Magic Dragon," Peter Yarrow, 1963

Endurance athletes are a funny lot. They do things that confound and confuse the rank and file. Men shave their legs, spend more time on a bike than in a car, leave a dozen pairs of sneakers on the front porch, go to bed at 9:00 p.m., wash down mountains of pasta with light beer, and when they do go out at night, hog the dance floor until closing.

I hate to stereotype (I'm an endurance athlete, and I never go to bed at 9:00), but I find it interesting to look at subcultures such as the folks who partake in extended athletic contests. You can generalize and be right more often than not. For instance, I could say that the "average" triathlete has a propensity for obsessive behavior–keeps a drawer full of race T-shirts, produces approximately 2.3 kids, drives a sport utility vehicle and has played golf less than ten times in his life–and I would be right in 61 percent of the cases.

But that formula doesn't work as well as it used to. Since the interest in long-distance events, and triathlons in particular, has grown, the diversity of the personalities has broadened considerably.

The reasons I participate differ greatly from those of Joe Bag-of-Donuts down the street. No one motivation is the "correct" one, although those of a more altruistic and deeply personal nature tend to offer lasting rewards.

The original triathletes were a different story altogether. Now that was a unique bunch: hard-training, hard-edged, hard-living characters. But, as the sport became more homogenized, they either disappeared into the sunset or altered their ways (for example, the original Ironman, Tom Warren, recently married).

But I enjoy being identified with this new cross-section of athletes, even if there are a few dweebs out there who walk around town with their race numbers plastered on their arms and legs.

The trick, it seems, is to remain a unique individual—march to a different drummer—while enjoying the comfort and security of the gang, if you wish. Not an easy task, but not impossible for those in the group that has come to think of an Ironman as a "Sprint."

IF YOU'RE REALLY A TRIATHLETE...

Several months ago, a leading men's magazine published a list of things a person should have accomplished by the time they reached 30 years of age. Reading the list, I realized that I was already halfway through my 30th year of existence. I knew I'd have to work extra hard if I was to complete the list before I turned 31.

Midway through the article, I gave up. I simply didn't have the time or desire to go out on a limb just to accomplish what society (and some overpaid, overweight writer) says I should.

That's when I decided to make a list for myself, my triathlete friends and you readers that we could relate to and have a fighting chance of completing. So the following are my suggestions for judging your progression as a triathlete based upon the number of races you've completed.

After finishing one triathlon, you should have:
- sworn never to do another one
- walked down a flight of stairs backwards because your legs were too sore to go forward
- told your friends that you and Dave Scott were good buddies
- signed up for swimming lessons at the YMCA
- decided that there must be some advantage to having more than one gear on your bike

After finishing three triathlons, you should have:
- bought a pair of ST shorts
- sneaked into the local hotel pool for a workout when the YMCA was closed
- asked a local cyclist what to do about those painful sores caused by your bike seat

- run at least ten miles without fainting, puking, or calling for a ride home
- asked someone not to smoke near you

After finishing five triathlons, you should have:
- considered shaving your legs
- told your boss that you were late for work because you were motor pacing (and felt good about it)
- told your spouse that you were late for dinner because you were time-trialing (and felt good about it)
- read at least one triathlon book

After finishing ten triathlons, you should have:
- considered dropping out of at least one triathlon
- had at least one bike crash
- told your friends that you and Scott Molina train together on occasion
- rinsed your cottage cheese at least once just to see how it tastes
- read the May, 1979 Sports Illustrated article on Tom Warren's Ironman victory

After finishing 20 triathlons, you should have:
- done at least ten 100-mile rides (centuries) without stopping for naps
- used one of your finisher T-shirts to wash the car
- considered moving to San Diego to train
- written a letter to Valerie Silk telling her you're dying of an incurable disease, and could she please let you into the Ironman

After finishing 25 triathlons, you should have:
- sworn you saw a shark when you were swimming in the ocean
- told your friends that Mark Allen is your third cousin
- learned what BLUSTS stands for
- gotten really mad at a race promoter
- shaved your legs and resisted the temptation to tell the person staring

at them that you just had knee surgery

After finishing 30 triathlons, you should have:
• thrown up in at least three races
• urinated in your wetsuit and felt good about it
• taken a trip to Boulder to train at altitude
• swam two miles without stopping

After finishing 40 triathlons, you should have:
• told your friends that you were a professional triathlete
• had your spouse threaten you with divorce on more than one occasion
• spent more on your bicycle than your car
• put more miles on your bike than on your car
• become blase about post-race massages

After finishing 50 triathlons, you should have:
• quit at least one job because they wouldn't give you the time to train
• obtained one form of sponsorship
• completed one Ironman distance race and lived to tell about it
• been a vegetarian for at least one year
• had the airlines lose your bike at least once

After finishing 100 triathlons, you should have:
• lost count of the number of races you've done
• talked about the "good ol' days" with your friends
• considered competing in the RAAM or the Western States 100
• sworn at least twice that you'd never do another triathlon
• had one hell of a good time and wouldn't trade it for anything...

THE MACHO SYNDROME

Sports is one of the key vehicles that have helped women attain equal status in our culture. But while the women's movement has "come a long way, baby," informal and institutional barriers to equality still exist. Even in our wonderful little world of triathlon, questions of sexism can be raised–the most significant of which is the issue of equal prize money.

It was only a few years ago that some sports were considered too strenuous for women. Now, both professional and amateur women are allowed to compete, usually alongside men. But consider that it took 22 Olympic Games for a women's marathon to be scheduled. The stodgy, bureaucratic power brokers of organized sports have for years stifled women's involvement, hiding behind the excuse that such events were far too difficult for women. More likely, it was a case of machismo.

This super-macho syndrome has not been an easy one for most men to shake, including me. Last year I entered Bend, Oregon's famous Pole, Pedal, Paddle race, a hybrid winter quintathlon that includes skiing and paddling. After I worked my way up from 120th place to 10th, I spotted the lead woman ahead of me, only a quarter mile from the finish line. An embarrassing yet successful last-minute sprint helped me save face from the ultimate shame of losing to a woman. Imagine how I felt when I found out the woman started five minutes behind me. Like I said, this has been tough for some men to handle...

Triathlons have been reasonably good to women, but probably not as good as women have been for triathlons. Females have provided a good share of the excitement in our sport over the years. Especially when you consider that during a period where only a handful of men have held down the top positions, more than a dozen women have shared top honors.

Even the television media continue to suffer from this testosterone tunnel vision. Recently, when one of the major networks chronicled a top female winning a prestigious ultra-distance race, they categorized her under the "excess-hormone" heading. And who can forget when one reporter in the same coverage remarked, "If most female triathletes are wide receivers, then this one is a left tackle." It seems like many of us have trouble treating women for what they are: athletes like anyone else.

It's also unfortunate that some of the best women triathletes have been tagged with certain stigmas. Erin Baker has been labeled a "terrorist" for standing up for her beliefs, Kirsten Hansen as a "Jesus Freak" for having a strong devotion to Christianity and the guts to talk about it, and Joanne Ernst as a "crybaby" for taking a stand on drafting. These women are some of the most considerate and caring people I know, and I admire them for their individuality.

The case of equal prize money for women has long been a point of contention. On one hand, you have those who have trouble justifying 50 percent of the purse to only 10 to 15 percent of the field. I remember a race not long ago that paid 15 deep and only had eleven women pros registered. (I tried to talk my mom and sister into racing.) Others will argue that the women work just as hard as the men, so why shouldn't they receive the same rewards? Indeed. What equal prize money would most likely do is encourage more women to participate and help legitimize them in professional sports–which helps women in general.

However, you feel about the issues, women have played a major role in the development of this sport and will continue to do so.

But as much as I admire their talents, I still dread the thought of... Never mind.

UNIQUE SUBCULTURE–IS TRIATHLON STILL JUST A FAD?

I was at a cocktail party the other night. It wasn't really a cocktail party, but more of a "basic pre-race invite a few pros, order a fruit & cheese plate for the benefit of the sponsors" type party. Having made the token minimum-but-effective round, I was carefully planning my silent exit when I overheard a "promoter type" bending the ear of "sponsor type." He said, "Triathlon really has become a Unique Subculture." Really, I thought, how and when did that happen? Is it good? I would have thought it was hoping to attain Legitimate Sport Status first (leaving behind the Underground Cult ranking).

Anyway, not having packed my dictionary on this trip, I wondered how Webster would have described Unique Subculture. I've heard it used in describing hippies, college fraternities and soldiers of fortune. So, for the sake of argument, I'll consider it a group or collection of individuals with their own distinct set of ideals, beliefs, rituals, clothing, jargon and style outside of society's norm. Okay, not bad.

With this is mind, the first step would be to figure out if any other sports have achieved Unique Subculture (U.S.) status. How about golf? Where else do you find lime-green polyester pants, but on the fairway? And the language; you don't find birdies, bunkers and bogeys in high-school spelling bees. But the ideals and beliefs are pretty mainstream. When you think about it, after all, a sport should leave you with enough energy to cut the lawn after a round of 18.

How about surfing? The ritual of throwing a surfboard off a cliff to bring big surf; the belief that searching for and finding perfect uncrowded waves is not unlike a Muslim's pilgrimage to Mecca for an true surfer; and the constant development of new and unique verbiage all give surfing a high U.S. potential.

Unfortunately, the clothing ruins it. In recent years, active-wear clothing manufacturers have so successfully developed, marketed and sold the "beach look" to millions of inlanders worldwide that local surfers have all, but given up trying to look any different from an Oklahoma City High graduate. In the United States, surfing is way too mainstream to be a real subculture anymore. Thanks, Hang Ten and O.P.

Bowlers? No, they drink plain-wrap beer. Fisherman? No, the only real ritual there is Saturday night bingo. Now, does Triathlon qualify for U.S. status? Let's have a look here.

Ideals and Beliefs
Triathletes believe that more is better. More mileage, more food, more expensive bikes. In most other sports (except the shot put and javelin) quality and speed are a factor.

Triathletes believe that to finish a race is a personal victory. In some other participatory sports, a personal record is the minimum to experience satisfaction. Score this round to the tri-heads as they are just a little different.

Who else would really believe that shaving the hair off your arms will make you run faster? Who else believes that $150 for a race entry is a good deal?

Ritual
Triathlon rituals. The carbo-loading party reminds me of an all-you-can-eat spaghetti night at the school gym–without the ever-present slide show. How about leaving your bike in the transition area overnight just because the Ironman does it? Let's get original, guys. The vaseline in the crotch is good, though. Whether or not you need it–a pre-race check list wouldn't be the same without it.

The clincher is body marking. Can the officials really read those things or is it just a long-standing ritual?

Clothing
In the beginning, you either dressed like a swimmer (green hair), a cyclist (European team jersey), or a runner (Boston Marathon finisher T-shirt). Now we have a look all our own. Part performance designed, part active-wear comfort and part "look at me" style. Triathlon clothing has transcended the specific market and spilled over into other buying segments. Fortunately, you don't have to live on the beach to be a triathlete.

Jargon
The language of triathlon is only partially developed, but unique. Hammer session, gear head, RDAC (recommended daily allowance of climbing) and duathlon (yick!) are all at least partially bred from triathlon rhetoric. Or maybe it was just that the conversation got boring during a STD (solid triple digit) bike ride.

Style
It's hard to say whether Triathlon as a sport has its own style. I know a few individuals in the sport who have it. I know others who don't. It's difficult, if not dangerous, to stereotype a collection of people with their own personal motives as having a single, common sense of style.

On the whole, the sport has in many ways developed a certain look, a certain feel. Some of that comes from the individual events that constitute triathlon. Make no doubt about it, our sport owes a lot to the history and make-up of swimming, cycling and running. Still more of triathlon's soul comes from the people themselves, especially those who aren't afraid to do things a little differently, to swim against the current.

The more we try to analyze, label, regulate, define and control, the more we become less of a Unique Subculture and more of a collection of three sports. Style is one thing, fad is another.

LIFE ON THE CIRCUIT

You must have heard at sometime or another that there is no such thing as a dumb question. Usually voiced by an inquisitive type, this truism is hard to argue with. Unless, of course, you have to smile politely, nod your head and answer yet another reporter's inquiries into, "What it's like to be a professional athlete?" That's okay though, it's when they stop asking you anything that you have to worry. Besides, they're just doing their job.

Another one of my favorites is, "What do you think you'd be doing if you weren't a professional athlete?" How should I know? It's the rare individual who ends up in a career he or she plans on since early childhood. And they usually become doctors or nurses. Actually, I did take one of those tests in high school that are supposed to tell you what kind of job you're best qualified for. I was slated to become a forest ranger.

For the benefit of the next journalist who really must know, the following is my version of "life on the circuit."

History

Since very early in the sport's history, there have been cash awards at races. Sometime in 1977 I competed in a race on Fiesta Island that had a one dollar entry fee. The entire gate (some 50 odd bucks) was awarded to the winner. Before he could accept it though, the organizers had taken the cash to buy beer for the awards, and graciously offered the suds in the winner's name.

Clearly, there was a little distinction between amateur and professional. Nobody earned a living off the sport until 1983. Even now there is not the type of separation between the ranks that there is in other sports. It bothers me when someone says, "Oh, you're a pro, you have an advantage." Barring genetic differences, everybody has the same rights and privileges when they make choices regarding their involvement in the sport.

Decisions
One of the most gratifying things you can ever hear is when someone says, "If I had to do it all over again, I'd do just what you are doing." That sort of falls into "The grass is always greener" category, but what it does say is that it's better to take a shot at realizing your athletic potential than to sit back in the old easy chair years from now and wonder, if just maybe...

Deciding to try and support yourself by competing in triathlons is a fairly heavy choice. To really succeed is even heavier.

Work Load
To people who say, "Man, I wish I had your job," my answer is, "No you don't." There are days I long for a desk job. To sit in a big leather chair, shuffle papers and flirt with the secretaries.

Actually, the work load of an elite-level triathlete is like that of most jobs–it's as hard as you make it. Success is often in line with the time and effort invested, whereas advancements in other careers can often get bundled up in politics and poor fortune, regardless of the individual efforts. I appreciate that about my chosen field.

Lifestyle
When it's good, it's good. When it's bad, it's bad. For instance, the opportunity to travel to new and exciting locations around the world is fantastic. But come October each year, like anything you max out on, it gets old. A 60-mile ride with friends on a warm sunny day is a blast. One hundred miles in the rain leaves a lot to be desired. Unfortunately, it's a package deal. Both are required for membership. The secret to success is enjoying as much of it as you can and realizing that every job has its undesirable aspects. All in all, earning a living by competing against others is a blast!

RIDING THE CREST

I've tried to make as many friends on my way up, because I know I'll probably lose half of them on the way down. People like to be around a winner; I certainly do. We must think that some of their success will rub off on us. In his book, Jim McMahon, quarterback for the Chicago Bears, tells a funny story about the time a fellow offered him $25,000 to stop by a party he was throwing. Unbelievable.

Actually, sincerity begets sincerity. Being a professional athlete does give you a chance to meet some very interesting people, but then, so does being a street sweeper. Whatever level of success you achieve, it's important to enjoy your achievements as well as your dreams.

The exorbitant salaries that professionals in other sports earn are derived from the fact that they are entertainers and marketing vehicles. Triathletes do not fall into the first category very easily because of the logistics of viewing the event. When triathlons are staged in large stadiums in front of thousands of spectators, million-dollar contracts will follow. I'll probably have retired to Ketchum, Idaho, to work as a forest ranger by then.

The Future

There is little doubt that the future for professionalism in triathlons looks bright. A dramatic downward turn in the economy could put a hold on these best-laid plans, but that would screw up everything else too.

What we are seeing is a move by everyone in the sport toward more professional behavior. That's good. As the bucks flow into triathlon, people in all areas are scrambling to get their share. That's not so good. Patience and hard work will reward the folks who are in it for the long run. And who could ask for a better job–getting paid to work at recreation that you'd probably do for free anyway? Certainly not I.

ONE MAN'S VIEW

The subject of women in sports often appears in newspapers and magazines, but I've never seen a story that discusses the current state of triathlon when it comes to the elite female competition. This brief discussion will not pose as a well-researched study on female athletes in our sport. It is (as always) only my personal opinion based on my years of experience in this sport. And, though I've never actually competed as a female (not even in disguise, as I've known some other jokers to do), I know the role of women in sport is a sensitive and volatile subject; especially explosive are the issues of equal prize money, separate starts and contribution to the sport.

There is no doubt that women have contributed greatly to triathlon and to sports in general. Even the most chauvinistic male will agree that sport has been a useful vehicle for women trying to advance the battle for equality, ever since the days when the term sportswoman was almost an oxymoron. But in triathlon, the gender battle lines have been drawn lately over the issues of equal distribution of prize money.

It's true that many people in this sport–men and women–worked hard for equal prize distribution. In the days immediately preceding the 1989 World Championship in Avignon, France, the U.S. men's team made it known to the race directors that it disagreed with the unequal prize structure; the organizing committee changed the system. That's one of the many examples. Yet the ringleaders of that particular crusade now find it ironic that the number of women pros has declined in recent years (while the pro men's field has grown exponentially).

The issue might be more palatable if as much money were offered today as once was. But prize purses have declined in recent years, and there have even been occasions when race organizers didn't have enough women in the pro field to pay out the allocated prize purse. Such situations, I think, undermine the argument that equal dollars attract more women.

Perhaps an insufficient number of younger women are attracted to this sport. Heaven knows the media has not always portrayed female triathletes in the best light. On the other hand, women who have been in triathlon for some years now feel pressure to call it quits. For some, this is social pressure to live a "normal" life; for some, this might be the maternal instinct calling.

Two of the longest and most successful careers belong to Erin Baker, 30, and Colleen Cannon, 31. Both have made it clear that they have accomplished what they set out to do, but more importantly, they feel a need to get on with the rest of their lives.

Does this imply that triathlon is not as viable a career option for a woman as it is for a man? The elite females are intensely competitive. One of the top women in this sport went so far as to say that her peers, as a group, were "all slightly neurotic." I don't know about that, but when you hear stories of one woman getting to the transition area at five AM just to get the best spot on the bike rack, you have to wonder if some of the women haven't taken it all a little too seriously.

I have tremendous respect for the accomplishments of Erin Baker, Colleen Cannon, Carol Montgomery, Karen Smyers and others like them, as well as for their overall contribution to the sport. It's the ones with their agent-driven, media-built images–who race only for fame, fortune and a boost to their entourage-fed egos–who bother me. But, as is the case with the analogous men, the public and the sponsors will eventually discover them for what they are.

A certain amount of irony laces the entire women's issue. In a time when the overall number of triathletes has decreased a bit, the number of women's–only races has exploded. A potential triathlete likes the idea of being able to race against other women without a bunch of macho guys clawing over her in the swim and springing ahead when she attempts to pass them on the run. I whole-heartedly support these races. If a race introduces more people to our sport, it's great.

Another bit of irony is found in the images of female triathletes. For instance, many people have been conditioned to think of Erin Baker as rough, driven and aggressive. But take away the game face, and you have as down-home and friendly a person you'll ever find.

Prize money or no prize money, the most progress is being made by the women you find in the front, middle and back of the age-group pack. They're the ones juggling a kid's soccer practice and trips to the store with careers and swim workouts. They embody the spirit of the sport and often wear the biggest smiles at the finish. Maybe the women pros can learn something from these amateur athletes. Life offers rewards during all of its seasons, if you just know where to look.

THE STRANGER–A PRIVATE LESSON IN VALUES

For many years, I got nervous on the night before important races. It was really the only thing that I disliked about being a serious competitor. I had tried a variety of tactics to free myself from these pangs of fear, but nothing really worked.

One day, prior to one of the Nice triathlons, I found myself in a conversation with a guy in his early 40s, an American who had seen the race on television and just had to try it once. There was a pause during our talk and the man turned to me and said very calmly, "Why are you so nervous? There is nothing to fear in a race, unless you are afraid of losing–and that is not the fear of a winner."

I didn't know what to say at first, but as the words sank in, I knew he was right. I wasn't afraid of getting hurt, though this course was somewhat dangerous, traversing steep hillsides in the Maritime Alps. Nor was I afraid of the pain that I knew would come during the race; I could deal with that as I did everyday in training, the same way we all deal with the pain–anyway we can. But when I really faced my pre-race fear honestly, it was true–I was afraid to lose. Afraid to disappoint my friends and family, to have to deal with the questions and excuses that a winner wouldn't be burdened with.

I asked this gentleman how he dealt with the fear of failure, an he said something that I'll never forget. "Triathlon is a game," he said, "and a game of little significance. Sure, you can earn your living from it, but in reality you're not going to starve if you don't win tomorrow. Your true friends don't give a hoot how you finish, as long as you race for the right reasons. You can never disappoint yourself so long as you finish with integrity and grace. And if your goals are shallow and self-centered; even winning every weekend won't ever give you happiness."

I asked how he had learned this philosophy of life and attained such a balanced perspective. "Years ago, when I was a young man," he said, "I found myself in the midst of a terrible firefight in Vietnam during what is now known as the Tet Offensive. I don't mind admitting that I was so scared I urinated in my pants. My body shook so hard I couldn't even talk. When I looked over at my buddy next to me in the foxhole, hoping for something... I don't know, courage, consolation–I saw that the left side of his head was caved in from the impact of a mortar shell. At that moment, a kind of strange calm came over me. It was part rage, part sorrow, part strength and part understanding. To this day, I have never felt fear like that. I compare any potentially harmful situation to war and I laugh at it. It's as simple as that."

He was right. Next to him, I felt trivial and my fears diminished. How can those of us who had the good fortune not to have experienced war, compare our fears to those who have? I envied him in a way. He knew the true meaning of life, since he'd been close to death in combat.

Fortunately, we can learn from people like him to help us put life in a proper perspective, but only if we have a mind to learn. When we exist from day to day in our own little worlds, it's easy to exaggerate trivial problems. Hell, it's part of human nature to manufacture challenges, simply to create a sense of achievement. But in the real world–the problems are far greater than finding new racing wheels by next week-end. In many places, safety, security and even survival itself is the order of the day. Keeping those realities in mind can give us strength of character, like it did to the guy in Nice.

The lesson I learned from him was that sport is a challenge, a pursuit of happiness. A race is an opportunity, not a cause for concern. We all face enough difficulty in just getting by, don't we? As we finished our conversation, he laughed quietly to himself and said, "When I wake up tomorrow, I'm going to look forward to a heart rate of 170 on the run. What doesn't kill me, only makes me stronger."

As he turned to leave, he paused and said with a wink, "It's not that life is short. It's just that you're dead so long."

THE SPORTS FAN

In the world of big-time professional athletics, 1993 was a year of good-byes.

We watched basketball great Larry Bird walk away with a nagging back problem and be denied a final season of deserved adulation from the crowds he had thrilled for so many years.

We watched baseball's most enduring legend, Nolan Ryan, take his farewell lap and almost make it all the way around until a shoulder injury sidelined him for the final month of his final season.

We watched Michael Jordan, arguably the most talented athlete to play any game, step away from it all while he was right at the very top. The King of the Hill just didn't want to play anymore.

And we watched solemnly while they laid Dodger pitcher great, Don Drysdale, to rest.

And in each case, I was saddened at first, then gradually, as I thought about it, pissed off. How could this be?

I was mad because Bird wouldn't be able to go out like Kareem and OJ with a damn parade in every city. A parade he deserved. I was mad at Ryan because he wouldn't be there for me to look at, marvel at, and say "Hell, he's seven or eight years older than me, and he can still bring it hot." I was mad at Jordan's retirement. here was a guy at the very pinnacle–I mean, if he went any higher on the scale, he'd need oxygen. And he just says, "No mas"?

As far as Big "D" goes, well, death is no picnic as it is, but to go early and leave a big hole to fill–it just plain sucks. Did I really have a right to be pissed off though? Was I wasting time and energy thinking about it, let alone writing about a couple of guys, regular humans off the field I might add, who quite simply were changing jobs? I was. But so were you.

Truth is, what self-respecting sports fan from Anywhere, USA, didn't cry when they watched Magic Johnson's retirement announcement? Any weekend warrior with half a heart can't think back to Lou Gehrig's farewell speech or watch Brian's Song without falling apart. And it's all because of selfishness.

We, you and I–John Q. Public, elevate these relatively normal folks to God-like status, paying enormous amounts to witness their great athletic skill. A skill they have individually honed by a lifetime of practice. And when the skill fades, or the individual tires of the medium and he decides to move on, we feel that something has been taken from us. Something that we hold dear, an anchor, an image, a hero. And heroes, like memories, are not easily replaced.

So we mourn the loss of our player, and we begin to elevate the next guy to build a relationship with his slam dunk or no-hitter. But is it fair? Is it fair to watch him sink 20-foot putts, one after another, or hit volleys as sharp as a Ginsu knife? Is it fair to ask him or her to give more than an honest 100 percent effort each time they enter the arena? The greats have collectively given us innumerable memories of athletic feats and raw courage to last for several generations. Should we expect their happiness too?

Jordan retired because he simply felt like it was time to move on–get on with his life. There are some people who claim that athletes like Jordan have almost become public property. If he had anything else to give, which of course he did, athletically, he owed his public whatever was left. But the basis for any athlete's decision to "Get on with his or her life" needs to be firmly grounded in the individual person's own mind and his own dreams and desires.

Of course, there are a variety of factors that go into his decision: "Am I more marketable if I quit before my inevitable decline? Are there still things that I want to accomplish in this sport? What lies ahead for me? What are my responsibilities to team members, family, friends, coaches?" But the biggest reason always should come right from where it all started: "Do I still love to play this game?"

And that, sports fans, is none of our business. Each and every athlete who partakes in any sport has to answer that question at some point in their career. They have to stand in front of the mirror and say, "Yo, how much do you still want it?" And no matter if they make $30,000 per game playing left field, or $300 for racing an Ironman, if they don't enjoy the simple purity of the activity–move on.

Maybe we expect too much in some areas and not enough in others. After all, sports legends are just people, aren't they? And for what they give us: memories, motivations, or just plain good entertainment (regardless of what they earn), don't we owe them a chance to play when they want, and walk away when they don't?

And, like in Drysdale's case, when they're really gone, be happy to have had a chance to witness magic in real life.

A Fan's Notes

I did something last weekend that I had done only once or twice before in my career. I watched a triathlon. And soon after the first competitors had left the water and taken off on their bikes it became obvious that every derogatory thing ever said about the spectator side of this sport is true. Viewing these races is not only borderline boring, it's hard. What the sport offers to the participant–safety, traffic control, security, the chance to be a hero–it takes away from the spectator. It's difficult to work around because of closed "athletes-only" areas, and often road closures make it hard to get out and see portions of the bike and run.

Unfortunately, in most cases, that's just the way it is. Triathlon has never pretended to be viewer friendly. The athlete's health and well being come first. After all, he or she is footing the bill; spectators never pay to watch. There just isn't that much to see. Or is there?

A few triathlons, primarily in Australia and France, have done the whole stadium thing, providing a great show for the fans. But these are not grassroots events, and they allow only a few elite professionals to compete. It's a vastly different event than what we see on an average Sunday morning in Anytown, U.S.A.

A few more have created loop-type courses that give spectators a number of opportunities to watch competitors as they come by. But these are somewhat of a hybrid and can suffer drafting problems. So for family, friends and curious onlookers who wish to catch more than a glimpse of the local out-and-back triathlon, what's the answer?

Here are my tri-fan survival guide suggestions:
1. Know the course ahead of time. This way you can strategically plot out your PVL (Primary Viewing Location).
2. Arrive early. Get a good parking spot, act like a volunteer, drink the coffee and mill around the transition area like you know what you're doing.

3. Offer to help. This may be the best way to actually be official and not feel guilty sneaking over the snow fencing. A race director can always use one more body.

4. Decide what you want to see. It's hard to see it all, so make a decision to, for example, watch just the start and first transition, or maybe park yourself at the bike turnaround and have time to jet back to the finish.

5. Get a press pass and take photos or write a story. It's not hard to get an assignment from your local paper. The regular sports writer certainly doesn't want to get up at 5 a.m., and most race directors welcome the press. Trust me.

6. Become a sports agent. They seem to be everywhere. How do they do it, anyway?

7. Take your binoculars, camera, camcorder, tape recorder and note pad. Keep them all going in all directions. You're bound to get plenty of material to check out later in the week.

8. Enter the race. You could actually pay your entry, do the swim easy, ride your own pace on the bike and walk the entire run–checking out the race as it goes by.

9. Watch it on TV. There was a lot of triathlon on TV this year, although the races that allowed drafting weren't really true triathlons.

10. Sleep in, pay a few bucks and go watch a ball game.

POETRY IN MOTION–THE MUSIC-ATHLETIC CONNECTION AND ST'S GREATEST HITS

Tennis great John McEnroe will often sit with a small club band playing rhythm or lead guitar along with his pal and fellow pro, Vitas Gerulaitis; Bob Marley could have played semi-pro soccer; two-time World Surfing Champion Tom Curren recently cut a live record in Australia, while ageless rocker Neil Young always takes his personal trainer on tour. When Kareem Abdul-Jabbar's house burned down, he lamented primarily the loss of his extensive jazz collection. Sammy Hagar had his own line of mountain bikes.

The cross-over between athletes and musicians has always been extensive. But that may only be the most noted of the parallels and intersections that exist between the two activities of music and sport.

On the surface they appear opposite, even conflicting. One is, for the most part, considered of a very physical nature, calculating, specific in movement, competitive and visual. Creating music, whether in song or use of an instrument, is a very specific and often technical from of physical movement. And who can say that watching a well trained team playing perfectly in sync is not a form of creative visual poetry? What do you remember about "Chariots of Fire"? The song or the true life story? For most people they are inseparable.

Yes, music and sport are indeed complimentary, if not divergent, means to balance one's life. Both are forms of expression, exemplified on one hand by a Springsteen concert and the other by whatever little tune pops into your head at mile 23 of the Marathon.

Try to imagine a baseball game without "The Star Spangled Banner." Or a dancer moving only to the applause of the crowd. Music makes you want to move–physically. And hitting a three pointer with ten seconds left in the quarter will naturally release a verbal song in response.

The most profound correlation, though, comes in the way each activity can alter one's mood, depending upon the type of music you play or the activity in which you participate. When I'm depressed, I lean towards a swamp level blues and a slow 20-mile trail run. Better moods attract a 60s rock and a crisp 40-mile ride on the Coast.

Does music affect the athlete in different ways than the non-physical?

Well, only in the fact that each individual reacts differently in any case. An athlete may choose to use music to put him or her in the proper frame of mind for training or competition. And in contrast, a musician will use physical training to develop the necessary skills to perform his or her music.

Just for the grins, here's my list of appropriate music for the various periods in a triathlete's life.

IN THE MORNING OF A HARD TRAINING DAY	
Group	*Album*
Sound Garden	Bad Motorfinger
Bruce Springsteen	Born to Run
Red Hot Chili Peppers	What Hits??

DURING A LONG, EASY RIDE	
Group	*Album*
R.E.M.	Out of Time
Jackson Browne	Pretender
Neil Young	Harvest

BETWEEN WORKOUTS	
Group	*Album*
Rod Stewart	Maggie May
Stevie Ray Vaughan	all albums
Bonnie Raitt	Luck of the Draw

AFTER A FLAT TIRE	
Group	*Album*
Eric Clapton	Unplugged
Junior Wells	all titles

RIGHT BEFORE A BIG EVENT	
Group	*Album*
Boston	Debut
Jimi Hendrix	Are You Experienced?
Pat Benatar	Best Shots

KIDS: THE REAL FUTURE OF TRIATHLON

I took my daughter to the park the other day. Like many two-year-olds, she is a real fan of a good swing. After settling into a rhythm, she says, "Higher, Daddy, higher." When I asked her why she wanted to swing higher, she replied, "Cuz it's more fun." Two swings over, I heard a little boy tell his mother that he wanted to go "just as high as that little blonde girl."

What prompts kids, or people of any age for that matter, to develop such opposing motivations for achievement? I've known people who compete for the pure and simple pleasure of just being out there–having a go of it, if you will. I've known others whose sole motivation to race comes from an inherent desire to beat someone. There are, of course, many others who are compelled by a combination of the two, as well as a host of other reasons that only they will ever know.

Many of us were instilled with a solid work ethic from a very young age. While this is good for climbing the corporate ladder and fueling a strong economy, it can certainly add an element of tension to a weekend softball game. We have become so "results" oriented that our recreation often takes on an air of stressful competition. Think about it. When did we all get so serious?

Our society puts so much pressure on winning that simple participation in the beauty of physical movement has little importance. I remember playing little league baseball and having to sit on the bench for whole games at a time because I wasn't good enough to play (or because my dad wasn't the coach). Kids are very impressionable at a young age. Such experiences can sour them on the politics of team sports for life. Why do parents have to live vicariously through their kids anyway?

It's difficult for people to change attitudes that they have harbored for so many years, but it's too late to set examples for the next generation of athletes and regular kids on the block. Goals are important. Sacrifice is important. Trying is important. But real success is achieved in the enjoyment of struggle.

There is a tremendous amount of politicking within the triathlon world that centers around the singular goal of acceptance to the Olympics. The argument is that an Olympic Triathlon will insure validity and a future to our sport. No one disagrees with this. But don't you think that the development of a strong youth program that instills the attitude of participation and enjoyment is equally, if not more, important to our own survival as a viable recreational opportunity?

Other than a semi-successful Ironkids program and the occasional "Kids Only" triathlon, what opportunities are there? The youth-oriented races aren't profitable and the kids don't buy a sponsor's products. But they will at some point. Let me ask the power brokers of our sport this: Are we not shooting ourselves in the foot by creating too many rules, too much emphasis on performance rather than participation, and too few opportunities for the youth of America to swim, bike and run?

Chapter 3

Rumors, Tales, Lies and Legends

Before CD-ROM, before video and voice mail, even before cheap magazines and books, there was the story, the tale of life's lessons. Morals and information of all sorts were passed down from generation to generation–not through the electronic media or written page, but by spoken word. And when told with conviction and enthusiasm, the themes became real, the legends believable. Children pondering a worldly choice could refer for guidance to the memory of a particular tale told upon a campfire evening.

Storytelling is now nearly a lost art, practiced by fewer and fewer people as we rely on Nintendo and Nickelodeon to teach our kids. And in the process, their creativity is sucked out, leaving a mental void to be filled with giant yellow birds and purple dinosaurs. Excuse me, but no matter how many times the letter X appears on Sesame Street, it is no substitute for the movie that plays in a child's head as a storyteller weaves an intricate tale.

I love a good story. Reading it, hearing it, telling it. It doesn't matter whether it's true. I'll file it in my scrapbook of memories, to pass on if the chance arises. Legends are gifts; heroes are valuable assets.

Sadly, though, some of our greatest sources of experience, our society's elders, are not sought out for their wisdom, but tucked away in some home where that fund of insight goes largely untapped.

Athletics is simply one more vehicle for experience. Create a story, embellish it, and at the appropriate time, speak the truth clearly, as you see it. Be someone's hero, if only your own.

TEE TALES–AN UNDERGROUND FASHION STATE-MENT

Consider the T-shirt. Once relegated to the undesirable task of retaining body odor and sweat within the confines of the undergarment, it's now a billion dollar media marketing tool. Think about it. We spend "gazillions of bucks" for a cotton T-shirt with somebody's logo on it, and proudly don that apparel because we want the world to know that we partake in the activity represented by the artwork on the back.

When I was growing up, I had to have one T-shirt for each sport that interested me (as an early cross-training enthusiast, there were more than a few). And I would wear those T-shirts with pride until they were threadbare. The shirts proclaiming an event were held in the highest esteem because they not only told the world I was a sportsman, but a competitor, too.

I'm not exactly sure how the T-shirt began its upward mobility. Certainly there was a time, maybe back in the 40s, that you just didn't walk around the streets in your undershirt. But a T-shirt is comfortable and as social pretensions of fashion subsided, "relaxed" garments became acceptable. How they came to be a walking billboard is anybody's guess. What a novel idea though? Slap a bit of color and design to an all-white T-shirt and whammo–wearable art!

Triathlon's contribution to this phenomena is the finisher's T-shirt. Coming in all shapes and sizes, from the neighborhood YMCA-triathlon to the elusive Ironman T-shirt, it's not only a way for us to display our talents, but a memento of our commitment to a particular event. At the same time, each individual triathlete has his or her own relationship with not only a triathlon finisher's T-shirt, but T-shirts in general. While I wear T-shirts more often than, say, dress shirts, I will often wear finisher's T-shirts that have nothing to do with swimming, cycling or running. But that is only because I overdosed on an all-encompassing approach to triathlons a while back. The average triathlete doesn't get to spend eight hours a day at it so he or she is stoked to put theirs on after work.

The shirt you pull from an over stuffed drawer to wear has a lot to do with your mood. If you're feeling particularly confident, you might wear your Sahara Desert Double Ironman shirt. But if you're not having a good day, you might choose the neighborhood 3K Fun Runner.

A T-shirt will also give you an indication of not only a person's interests or moods, but his finer points (or lack thereof). For instance, if a 300 pound woman is wearing a shirt from the NCAA gymnastic championships, she probably shops at Goodwill.

The most valuable shirts are the oldest and most broken-in ones. Scott Molina must have a collection of 500 old race shirts he has saved over the years. His favorite is faded orange with rips in the sleeve and has the word "RUN" in black letters on the chest. He got it in 1972, and has logged literally thousands of miles running in it. T-shirts will appreciate with time, especially if they are kept in reasonably good condition. The more obscure the event, the better.

I haven't managed to hold on to as many as Molina, but the flagship of my small, but enigmatic collection is from a tennis tournament in 1973 entitled, "The Battle of the Sexes." It featured Björn Borg vs. Evonne Goolagong, and the logo on the back was really cool.

The T-shirts that I have dispersed with have gone to some interesting locales. I used to give some of them to my grandparents when they lived in a retirement community. All the old codgers got a kick out of my grandpa doing his daily walk in a T-shirt from a moto-cross race or a surf contest. Quite a few others have found their way to villages in Mexico. I have a classic photo of a 5-year-old boy wearing a T-shirt that says, "Diamond Triathlon of the Stars–Where your dreams come true." Quite a cultural oxymoron.

If you can't seem to find an appropriate place to bequeath your extra shirts and can't bear to use them to wash the car, try making a quilt out of them.

Better yet, have someone else make one for you (Tee-Quilts, (916) 989-1414) with your stock.

T-shirt swaps used to be kind of popular at races, but too many Tri-heads were unable to part with the one piece of physical validation that remained after the pain went away, and the race photo faded. When you think about it, it would be hard to explain that you really didn't complete the race on your back, but you met a fellow who did– it used to be his shirt! Much too complicated.

The greatest irony of all surrounding T-shirts, though, is the much maligned polyester blend tank top that our fathers wore, and we laughed at. Appropriately called "the beater", it is now, fittingly, the fashion statement of the underground grunge look. Could it be that we have become the people our parents warned us about?

THE GOOD, THE BAD AND THE UGLY

The phone rang. My wife says, "It's C.J. at *Triathlete*. He wants to know where your article is." I had already used every excuse possible, including thermonuclear explosion of my typewriter. I had to go for the "big one" this time. "Tell C.J. I have writer's block. He'll understand," I called out. The reply was as subtle as a cold shower–"You've got 24 hours, period!"

Actually, it does become difficult to be original, witty and informative every month. A quick call to my literary mentor, triathlon journalist Mike Plant, was in line. "Just put it down on paper, man, don't force it. Open your eyes an ears and let it flow out," he said.

I looked around. A poster from an old sailing regatta–maybe a piece on traveling or off-season diversions? No, bad time of year. A Power Bar wrapper on the table suggested yet another nutritional sampler. No way! On the radio a classic instrumental and movie title track from the 60s cranked. And there it was. I'll do a piece on triathlons "The Good, the Bad, and the Ugly"!

The Good
1. Your first ride on a new bike. It doesn't squeak, it shifts like a dream and you could eat breakfast off the bottom bracket it's so clean.

2. Your boss at work hears that you did a triathlon last weekend and from then on he seemed to show you just a little more respect, even though he never mentioned the race.

3. Your friends are talking about how they have trouble falling asleep at night. You smile to yourself because you can't recall the last time you saw ten PM on the clock.

4. You're finishing your first triathlon, and even though you said you would only do one, you instinctively realize that this is the beginning

of a much bigger commitment. But you feel good about it even though you don't know why.

5. You order two dinners at the restaurant and when the waiter gives you a "he must be bulimic" look because you're too thin to eat this much, you guiltlessly ask for extra rice.

6. You're out to a pre-dawn run and the stillness of the morning is inspiring you. When an overweight tourist stops to ask directions to a donut shop, the cigarette smoke escaping out the small window opening, he ends the conversation with "you're a better man than I." You turn and start running again and think to yourself, he said it, I didn't.

7. You go over to your 20-year high-school reunion and when an old flame says, "You haven't changed a bit," you reply, "Oh, well, I've lost a few pounds."

8. When you do your tax return, you can honestly write off things you never thought possible without a trace of guilt. Hey, you're a pro tri-athlete, aren't you?

The Bad

1. You total up how much you spent on massage last year, and for a brief moment, wonder if the expense was a bit vain.

2. Your newly oiled bike chain has just imprinted a nice "railroad tracks" graphic on your velour car seat.

3. You walk into a local bar for a beer, forgetting you have your shorts on, and a Hell's Angel won't stop staring at your shiny, smooth legs.

4. It's the night after a long race and you pop a newly formed blood blister on your toe with a sterile needle. Unfortunately, the blood gets all over your wife's white satin couch. You suddenly realize you will be sleeping on that very same couch for the next three nights.

5. You read a proposed rule by some power hungry idiot that has us all on the same type of bike, wearing the same shoes, etc., and you ask yourself, "Am I living in a democracy, or has America gone socialist?"

The Ugly

1. Five minutes before the start of a race, you rub some Vaseline on your more-than-sensitive body parts and realize that a hundred people are staring at you, wondering just what it is that you're doing with your hand in your pants.

2. You can't close your T-shirt drawer because it's crammed with race T-shirts you've never worn. Your wife won't dare throw one away, because the last time you caught her dusting with a particularly ragged one, you likened the situation to sneezing on an American flag.

3. On the way home from a race, you stop by a 7-11 to get a cold drink, and when the clerk sees the numbers on your arms and legs, he glances at the "wanted" pictures next to the cash register to check any resemblance.

THE CHALLENGE–A SHORT STORY

The phone rang. At first Trevor thought he must have been dreaming–it couldn't be morning already. He had just gone to sleep, or so he thought. It rang again. Trevor swore at what he thought was an unwelcome alarm clock. Then, with the sleep leaving his dream-filled head like a thick fog burning off in a spring morning, he realized that the disturbance was the phone ringing.

Trevor reached for the receiver and glanced at the clock while he tried to guess who would be calling at 3:15 a.m. Any call at that hour had to be a joke, a wrong number, or a death in the family. It couldn't be good. His fears were realized when his father told him that his lifelong pal and former neighbor, Billy Robbins, had been killed by a drunk driver earlier that evening. Trevor's heart sank as his father recounted the story of the accident and Billy's struggle to survive on the operating room table–the massive internal injuries finally dousing his incredible will to live.

As Trevor's dad explained how they found the note in Billy's wallet requesting immediate notification of two individuals upon his death, he thought of the similar note in his own wallet. He recalled how he, Billy and Jack "the Rabbit" Wilson had sealed their fates nearly 20 years ago. Back then, the three of them were only days away from high school graduation. Each had his own plans for the coming fall, and they somehow knew–instinctively–that even though they had spent the better parts of their childhood hanging out together, their lives would go separate ways very soon. Trevor would go to college, Billy to his father's business and Jack to the jungles of Southeast Asia.

The three had decided to justify their existence and celebrate their own rites of manhood by attempting a feat of athletic endurance that all of them considered extremely difficult, but not insurmountable.

Of the three, Jack "the Rabbit" Wilson had, by far, the most athletic ability. Ironically, though, he had never played on a varsity team while in school. Nobody knew exactly why, but some of the upperclassmen told a tale of politics and corruption in the school's football program. The same coaches who had recruited Jack away from his rough neighborhood on the other side of town would ultimately drive him away for his failure to play by their rules.

Trevor's ability was average, but he worked hard and lettered in track and basketball. Of the three, he seemed to enjoy sports the most.

Billy lacked the physical skills of Jack and Trevor, but made up for it in guts and determination. Weighing a good 30 pounds less than most of the other guys in his class, he often took a beating, but he seemed to gain inner strength each time he was abused. Maybe that explained his refusal to die from injuries that probably would have killed others instantly.

They decided that each of them would write out the most difficult workout he could think of within his favorite sport, then they would put the sheets of paper into a hat and draw in turn. Each boy would have to complete his workout within eight hours.

They drew straws to see who would pick first. Jack won. He reached into the hat and pulled out all three sheets. Quietly, Jack walked to a window and looked out. Then he slowly turned around and said, "I'll do each one consecutively and finish under 24 hours."

"Jack, you have no idea what those papers contain," Billy replied. "I know my workout was outrageous by itself, and Trevor here has a gnarly streak in him. I'm sure his is no picnic."

Jack walked back to the window and said, "It doesn't matter. The three of us will do it together."

The gauntlet had been thrown down. Trevor submitted with, "OK, as long as we can do it in one day. Let's just open the sheets of paper and check first."

But Billy sealed the agreement when he said, "No, we all agree to do it, no matter what it is, no matter what it takes, even if it kills us!" There was a seriousness to his voice that the others hadn't heard before, as if Billy sensed both the difficulty and the opportunity in the challenge at the same time.

Trevor agreed and took the three sheets from Jack. Each boy opened one and read it aloud. "Workout one: ride your bike to the top of Mount Windswept, 178 miles. Workout two: run to the top of Cochise Pass, 37 miles, including 7,000 feet of climbing. Workout three: swim across Laredo Lake, over four miles."

They couldn't believe that they had chosen three different sports, all individual efforts, all endurance oriented and all in the same geographical region. Jack broke the silence. "We go next Monday, the day before I have to report to boot camp," he said.

Trevor hung up the phone and forgot about trying to get back to sleep. He had too much to do, too much to think about, and he had to find Jack. The note in his wallet, the one they found in Billy's and most likely the one that Jack had kept with him all these years meant the promise had to be kept, just as they had agreed.

Soaking his head under the steaming shower, Trevor once again reflected on that big day, 20 years ago. It had not seemed that difficult at first. The bike ride took close to ten hours and, fortunately, their early start and the northern latitudes' long days left them with enough daylight to get a good portion of the run in before dark. Still, it was getting tough, and they definitely had not trained for it.

They had finished the run with flashlights and then stood on the edge of Laredo Lake–staring out into the cold, dark, calm waters.

There are probably only a handful of moments during a lifetime in which people have a chance to view their past and future very clearly and very much at the same time. For these kids, this was one of those moments.

Billy looked at Jack, who didn't say a thing. Jack just took off his shoes and shirt and stepped into the lake. He swam about 20 yards out, stopped and said to the others, "It's just like a glorified game of Marco Polo." Whereupon he yelled, "Marco!" and not expecting a reply, swam away.

Trevor and Billy watched in disbelief as Jack swam calmly yet deliberately through the cold Laredo Lake waters. He had started in the general direction of the far end of the four-mile-wide lake. But when he was no more than 200 yards offshore, he disappeared into the moonless night, enveloped by the surface fog that seemed determined to swallow anything that disturbed its tranquil beauty.

The two looked at each other and knew they had no choice, but to follow. It was a decision only partially prompted by concern for Jack, now somewhere on his way toward the far shore and–they hoped–completion of the 200-mile-plus endurance trek. No, they knew that what they faced was a deeply personal challenge that was as important for them individually as it was for each other.

It was two decades since that memorable night and Trevor found himself alone in his bedroom, still shocked by the call from his dad, detailing Billy's death earlier that evening. He walked to his dresser and reached for his wallet. Without opening it, he walked out into the early morning stillness, across the yard and into the barn. Fortunately for him, Marie and the three kids were away for the weekend, but still he felt a sense of peace in the barn and wanted to think for a minute.

Would it still be there in his wallet after all these years, crumpled beneath credit cards and pictures of the kids when they were too young to walk–and to understand things like this? Sitting on a flattened basketball, he opened the wallet and searched. There it was...

yellowed and barely readable. He recited the oath he had taken 20 years ago:

"Upon the death of any of the three of us (Trevor, Billy and Jack), the surviving two parties (or one) will recreate the events of the day that each participated in on June 30, 1970. Nothing is to be omitted and the only stipulation is that the time for the three events must be faster than originally recorded. If that time is not achieved on the first attempt, then subsequent and consecutive attempts must be made until the record is broken. Failure to do so will be considered disrespectful to the deceased party and will otherwise render our lives useless.
Agreed in full:
Trevor Jack Billy
July 1, 1971"

Trevor's father was an attorney and had helped them write the agreement on the day after their original adventure, thinking it was a boyhood prank, without meaning or commitment.

And now, Trevor sat contemplating the same. Was it a hollow promise made by a couple of kids heading in different directions or was there more to it? He reflected on the times over the past years when he had started to let himself get out of shape, but each time had strangely bounced back into his routine.

For the first time, he was beginning to realize that this little agreement in his wallet, the adventure of 20 years ago and, more importantly, his childhood commitment to his two buddies had helped shape his life. These events had given him something to hang on to, like a life raft that was always there in rough areas—whether you used it or not. In past years, the knowledge that he was in shape for a reason, and so were his buddies, was enough.

Suddenly he felt better. Still troubled by Billy's death, Trevor was nevertheless better now that he had a clearer picture of his youth and a knowledge that he had to find Jack. They had to return to Mt. Windswept, Cochise Pass and, ultimately, Laredo Lake.

Finding Jack would be tough. While Trevor and Billy had tried to stay in touch, exchanging Christmas cards and the annual phone call, Jack had disappeared nearly twelve years ago and was not the type to write post cards.

Glancing around the barn (the sun beginning to shine through cracks in the wall), Trevor's eyes rested on his old bicycle. Rusted out and probably beyond repair. He smiled when he saw the ancient swim goggles hanging from the handlebars, with spider webs spun from lens to strap. He tried to remember whether he had worn goggles the night they swam across Laredo Lake.

Trevor and Billy had been trying to swim close to each other, stopping occasionally to yell for Jack. The wind had picked up, clearing out the fog, but stirring the lake's surface into a 2-foot chop. They had been swimming for over and hour and still hadn't seen Jack or their destination on the other side of the lake. At one point Billy had thought he heard someone yell, "Marco!" in the distance, but had written it off as the wind and his own tired brain.

Finally, after nearly two hours of swimming, Trevor spotted the shore. The sun was beginning to rise in the East, casting dark gray shadows on the choppy waters. Billy and Trevor were treading water, contemplating how they were going to make the last half-mile–both of them were so fatigued that they felt they might cramp and drown right then and there.

"If you two wimps waste any more time, we'll never make the 24-hour time limit." It was Jack; he'd doubled back and snuck up on them.

Trevor and Billy were relieved to see Jack, but weren't concerned about the time limit as much as they were their own well-being.

Jack spoke again, "We set a goal and we can achieve it. It's less than a half-mile, the sun's coming up and we've got fifteen minutes left. Do this and I promise you'll never forget it! Vamanos, amigos."

Trevor laughed to himself as the animals in the barn began to awaken, and he thought about the three of them lying on the beach at the far side of Laredo Lake–totally spent from exhaustion, but filled with pride, accomplishment, and camaraderie. Then he felt someone staring at him from the barn door. Turning around he heard a familiar voice say, "I got two new bikes, some awesome running shoes, and these goggles with built-in night-vision capabilities. You'd better be in shape, pal. Billy would be pissed if we had to do this more than once to break our record." Trevor, shocked at first by Jack's sudden appearance, simply said, "Piece of cake–if I don't have to wait for you again."

A SMALL TOWN INTERLUDE–THE PIT STOP

I sat on the curb in front of an old rickety store, gulping the last of who knows what that was fermenting at the bottom of my water bottle. I was midway through a solitary 140-mile ride and fresh out of Cytomax, PowerBars, courage and testosterone when I stopped in this "one horse town" to rest my weary bones. (And besides, I had to take a leak.)

I don't know if this place had name, but it definitely had a feel. You know how it is. You arrive in a particular place and suddenly your mind is flooded with all sorts of intangible sensations that give you a sixth sense of your surroundings. As soon as I got off my bike in this "miles from nowheresville town," I felt it. A sense of simplicity and innocence permeated the air.

Two teenage boys were hanging out in the store gawking at pictures from Playboy that they had slipped inside a Popular Mechanics magazine so the store manager wouldn't catch them and toss them outside into the stifling heat. After a few minutes, they wandered out and looked at my bike. "Where'd ya come from?" asked a tall, rangy looking kid with a half-dozen pimples on his chin. Then "How many days it take ya?"

"Four hours," I replied and then showed them my computer with the time and distance display to verify my claim. Visibly impressed, but unwilling to concede anything, this stocky kid with unlaced high-top sneakers said, "That doesn't sound too hard on a 10-speed racing bike like that. How much does it weigh?"

Sensing that this interlude was predestined and some type of learning opportunity, I parried back. "Hey, wanna try it? I bet you could motor right up that big hill." I pointed to a nasty-looking driveway with a 20 percent grade and said, "Your buddy and I will just sit here and finish our Cokes. Come on, go for it."

So the kid climbed on and immediately had a problem with the strange looking pedals, not to mention the fact that the seat was six inches too high and I had slipped it into the 53/12 gearing. Nevertheless, he rode off fearlessly toward the big hill. I sat quietly with his rangy friend and watched as he zigzagged up the beastly hill. "So," I asked the rangy kid, "what do you guys do for fun around here?" He answered. "Not much, really. Look for crawdads down by the creek sometimes. My friend has a Nintendo, but it's busted right now."

"How about sports?" I asked. "Who's your favorite basketball player?" "Oh, I don't really do much sports," he replied, "I think Bon Jovi shreds, don't you? added the stocky kid who had returned a few moments ago.

Can We Make a Difference?
It was at this instance that I thought to myself, "What's happening here?" These two kids seemed to be fairly typical teenagers from Anytown, USA. Still, there was something wrong, something missing. Maybe I was just prejudging the two boys because their hero was a rock and roll singer with skinny arms and pasty skin instead of Magic Johnson or Larry Bird. Or maybe I felt sorry for them because the boredom of this town might cloud their prospects for what society has labeled as "success." I don't know.

The fact is, there are probably millions of kids just like these two whose primary influences are not family, education and sport, but MTV, Nintendo and peer pressure. Is it society's fault? Is it the parents' fault? Or am I rambling on about nothing? As the saying goes, "Kids will be kids."

As I climbed back on my bike for the next 70-mile stretch, I couldn't help, but think that with all the talent, power, money and influence in the sport of triathlon—what is our contribution? Do we set a good example? Can we make even a small difference? Hey! Where's my bike computer?

BITS AND PIECES FROM THE FIRST 100 ISSUES

One of the cliches I often heard as a kid, but never fully understood, was: "It's the little things that count." Adults were always telling me: "It's the less-than-monumental moments that stay with us," or "Though they seem inconsequential at the time, the little things as a group will make up your strongest memories." If you think about it, it's true. Sure, we hold onto life's heavy events, but quirky little tidbits, both unique and unexpected dominate our memories.

With that in mind, I sat down to recall a few of those quirks, using the early issues of *Triathlete Magazine* to prod my memory. Looking back through these pages made me laugh and frown and just plain wonder what the heck we've all been doing for the past ten years.

Things I wish I had a picture of:
1) Carl Thomas sweeping up the transition area after the first USTS in 1982.
2) The look on a young Kenny Souza's face the first time he came to San Diego to run with the big boys.
3) Colleen Cannon and me winning a dance contest after a 1983 USTS race.
4) The pack of 20 pros riding together in the 1987 Bermuda Triathlon.

Best dressed:
1) Team J David, with the American-flag skin suits we wore at the 1983 Nice Triathlon.
2) The guy who did the 1982 Ironman in a spandex full-length bodysuit because he thought it would keep him cool. Can you imagine swimming 2.4 miles with long sleeves and legs?
3) Cowman, whenever he races.

Things I'm glad there are no pictures of:
1) The time I had to stop and relieve myself during the run at Nice with only four or five hundred people watching.

2) "Borrowing" two stretch limos to cruise around after the 1984 Bahamas.

3) Colleen Cannon and me winning a dance contest after a 1983 USTS race.

Most spectacular disqualifications:
1) Jacqueline Shaw at an early World's Toughest Triathlon, for failing to come to a complete stop at a stop sign. As a result, she had to forfeit the $10,000 first place award she had won.

2) Erin Baker at a mid-80s Nice Triathlon, for taking a cup of water from an unofficial aid-station spectator. It only cost her first place and about ten grand. Of course, nobody ever violates that rule!

3) Patricia Puntous at the 1986 Ironman, for drafting. She was told about the DQ after she had run her heart out to win the race.

Best printable quotes (without pissing someone off):
1) "If there would have been prize money, I would have run him over."–Scott Molina, on why he stopped to help Dave Scott after a bike crash during the 1985 Ironman Japan.

2) "Within five years, all of you guys should be making big bucks."–Larry King, executive director of the Association of Triathlon Professionals, at a 1983 meeting.

3) "Where are all the race-director groupies?–Jim Curl, co-founder of the Bud Light USTS, as he and I arrived in Atlanta for a race.

Worst dressed:
1) Anybody who wears a racing-type swimsuit anywhere other than on a race course.

2) Guys who train in teardrop-shaped aerodynamic helmets.

"Which way did he go?" award:
1) Me, for getting lost–not once, but twice–at the 1990 Japan Ironman, a course I had done four times before.

2) John Hellemans of New Zealand, for finding a way to cross the finish line from the wrong direction at a race in Sydney, Australia.

Best excuses for dropping out of a race:
1) "I want to have babies someday."–Julie Moss, 1987 Ironman.
2) "A hundred years from now, who's going to remember who won this race?"–unidentified.
3) "I had to look down at my legs to make sure they were still there."–unidentified athlete, at the 1982 Malibu-Tri (regarding the 1.5-mile swim in 58 degree water without wetsuits).

Greatest vindications of triathlon:
1) When cyclists started using aerobars after initially calling them "tri-geek" bars.
2) When cross-training became a household word.
3) When tri-phenom Lance Armstrong became one of America's premier cyclists.

Best reasons to be a triathlete:
1) You can eat a lot.
2) You don't have to hang out with runners and talk about splits, PRs and air soles.
3) You don't have to hang out with cyclists and talk about gear ratios, derailleur technology and famous European mountain passes.
4) You don't have to hang out with swimmers and stare at the walls.

Best time to admit you're a triathlete:
1) When clearing customs.
2) When you're getting pulled over by a cop.
3) When a group of Hell's Angels are making fun of your shaved legs.
4) When ordering your third stack of pancakes.
5) Any time it will get you a discount.

Best quote during a race:
"Hey, you guys want to go long today?"–Paul Huddle, Ironman Canada, when he caught Ray Browning and me early in the bike.

THE PLAYER

The player told the cab driver to pull over next to the wharf. He wanted to look a the tidal currents before driving to the dock and the place they called Ground Zero. He got out of the car and walked over to the edge of the bay. Looking out beyond the seedy cannery district and past the anchored tuna fleet, he reflected on his life: how it had become so bizarre, so unusual in such a short time.

Only six months ago, the player had an office on the twenty-third floor in one of the ominous buildings which loomed over the water across the bay–home to hundreds of multinational conglomerates which, from his vantage point, provided a strange reflection of light on the cold, dark water on this moonless night.

He had left his small apartment early this time, somehow knowing that he would require extra time to prepare himself for tonight's competition. Something inside had also told him to take a cab and avoid having the unnecessary baggage of a vehicle. The player still sat on the deck, knowing he had plenty of time until the midnight start, and so allowed himself a long moment to ponder the unpredictable twists of fate that had led him to this moment.

Less than two years go he relished his job as an account executive with a large and prominent public relations firm. He loved everything about the job and his life: the expensive cars, the competition of the business, the singular focus on nothing more than the bottom line. But one day, something snapped and the excitement was gone; the thin veil of his transparent existence had left as quickly and effortlessly as a whisper in the wind.

The player looked elsewhere for thrills, knowing instinctively that he was a person fueled by the dare of insurmountable odds and powered by the passion of the hunt. If he couldn't get this fix in the world of commerce, he would have to find it in another pursuit.

Hunting didn't interest him, he'd done it with his buddies, but had a hard time killing animals simply for sport. For a time, he raced cars and motorcycles, but found it very cost prohibitive, especially with his all-out style of driving. He even ventured for a while into the underworld of illicit activity. And even though gambling and bookmaking seemed harmless, he saw first hand what lawlessness does to the hearts and minds of otherwise good men. The circles in which he traveled in this dark realm were the same he was due to see later tonight.

But it was running that finally fueled the flames of his soul.

He had been stuck in traffic one Saturday morning on his way to a meeting. After sitting motionless in his car for nearly 15 minutes, he got out and walked to the traffic light and asked the policeman what the holdup was. At the corner he encountered a wall of humanity running down the middle of the street. An endless parade of people, of all sizes, shapes and colors, ran past wordlessly in an endless procession. The police said they wouldn't all be past for another 20 minutes or so, and the road would be closed for at least that long.

At first the player was furious with the delay. But, gradually he justified the wait with the knowledge that these people had just as much right to the roads as his big BMW and collectively contributed less pollution than the dozen cars waiting with idling engines to get past the road block.

Then something strange happened. The player felt himself being pulled into the sea of runners. Like a magnet, he was sucked into the group, and there was nothing he could do about it. One moment he was just another angry, self-centered executive late for a client meeting, the next he was running down the road in slacks and dress shoes with a thousand other athletes.

It was the strangest thing the player had ever felt: No longer was he in control of his actions. After the first block, he was gasping for air. The second found him noting the pain in his feet. On the third block, a huge smile came to his face and he felt a weight lift from his shoulders. He knew he had found a new challenge in his life–running.

He ran five miles that morning, unconscious of his bloody toes, chaffing crotch and screaming muscles. It was only when he attempted to sprint across the finish line in his street clothes (hoping to beat the older, but fit looking guy he had been pacing off of), with no number, no race bib, and not even looking like he belonged, that he realized what had happened. It had been a dream-like sequence, but the player knew it was real and he embraced it.

Later, he hitched a ride home with a girl from the office whom he had recognized, but decided to leave his car where it stood–it became a monument to his past, to a life he no longer lived. The leasing company could have it back, he told himself, he had little use for the leather interior now.

The following weeks were filled with the excitement of the change that consumed his life, and he rejoiced with the pain of training himself into shape. The player didn't mind the training, he even enjoyed parts of it, but knew inside that what he was after was a race. For him, preparation was important, but nothing would take the place of the primitive battle in the athletic arena. It didn't matter that at first it would be for a top age-group finish in some po-dunk 10K, he would end up the stakes soon enough.

And now, staring into the black, polluted and shark-infested waters in which he would swim later that night, he couldn't help, but allow himself just a while longer to try and make some sense of the events that changed him from a weekend jogger to a fierce and menacing competitor in a very dangerous, high stakes sport.

At first the player was satisfied with top placings in his age group, at least that was enough to satisfy his insatiable need to compete. But even after a few overall victories (which surprised even him given the fact that his athletic talents were always good, but never world class) it became apparent that it wasn't the accolades of success that motivated him, but the process of getting to the victory stand. He knew that winning, for him, was not what he strived for. It was the thrill of the hunt; of the moments of intense competition when he felt most alive, when nothing else mattered, but putting himself just a step closer to the brink of physical collapse. He knew instinctively the danger in racing to the extreme like this, but the player wasn't concerned about "lifelong fitness," he was an adrenaline junkie, plain and simple.

The 10Ks gave way to marathons. The marathons turned into 100 milers and somewhere along the way he discovered a format that fit his competitive drive like a glove. Triathlon.

But even his life in triathlon took a strange and dark twist one day. As a result, he found himself here and now, only a few hours away from another battle in this inner city multi-sport madness where victory meant more than a finisher's medal.

Benjamin woke and he woke hard. His undershirt and shorts were soaked with sweat, the kind that comes after a deep and disturbing sleep punctuated with dreams too real to ignore, but too strange to believe. It had been this way lately, frantic days and restless, dream-filled sleep.

Last night, he had the same recurring dream that placed him in a strange life-or-death athletic contest centered around a seedy, underworld crowd and a darkened wharf location. The dream is almost always the same.

Benjamin doesn't know how the dream story will end, but he surmises that it might be a combination of Russian roulette, rollerball and devil-take-the-hindmost.

They say that dreams can teach us many things and that they are often a strange juxtaposition of recent events–or future occurrences. But

Benjamin didn't really pay too much attention to the details of his dreams. He was a busy guy right now with an executive-level job, a demanding girlfriend and an exercise program intended to support both.

But there were too many parallels, too many comparisons between his day-to-day existence and his nighttime episodes to dismiss.

Benjamin was a driven and competitive player, a man who not only thrived on competition, but needed it like a junkie's fix. He wasn't proud of it, but he seemed helpless to change. And lately, his choice of competitive venues had gotten him into deep trouble. Deals had gone sour because he had tried to bargain for that one last point, giving him the feeling of victory in corporate negotiation. His quest for dominance had wreaked havoc in his personal relationships and it was only his athletic interests that tolerated his competitive drive.

In Benjamin's dream, the player also suffered from a dysfunctional drive. Strangely enough, it seemed acceptable to the society in which he lived, just as Benjamin's own real world had tolerated his interest for victory, so long as the bottom line was achieved.

As he dressed for work, it was this particular point that Benjamin focused on. Was he indeed suffering from a psychological malady or was he simply a by-product of a society that condones intense, results producing competition, rewarding the victors with numerous accolades? After all, didn't what's-his-name, the left fielder, just sign for $6 million a year?

Driving to work, Benjamin decided to take the coastal route. He had no idea why, but he eventually found himself down by the old wharf where the tuna boats unloaded their nightly catch. He had never been to this part of town before, but it all seemed very familiar, disturbingly so. He parked his car near an old wooden dock and walked over to the sea-wall. It was relaxing, sitting there in the mid morning sun watching the fishermen–until he realized that this was the very spot that his dream ended each night when he awoke in a panic. He would always be standing right here, looking out over the harbor, waiting for some athletic contest with life-or-death circumstances to begin.

Benjamin was both terrified and fascinated at the same time. How could he have known to come here? What was the significance of the impending competition? Was there a parallel to his own real world that he didn't fully understand? What was the message in all of this?

Just as his head spun with ideas and concepts, he was yanked back to reality by the ring of his cellular phone. It was his office. Where was he? He was supposed to be at a very important meeting this morning, but had completely forgot. His secretary spoke in a quiet, dull tone and calmly informed him that the meeting had gone bad. The clients had walked out and his partner had jumped out of the window of the 23rd floor only a few minutes later. His boss wanted him to get over to the clients' office right away and see if he could patch up the deal. Yes, it was too bad about his partner, but life goes on and business is business.

Benjamin got back in his car and began to drive downtown. Like a bolt of lightning, it all became very clear. He stopped his car in the middle of the street and got out. Running slowly along the water's edge, his metamorphosis had begun. He never liked the 23rd floor anyway.

RUMORS, LIES AND TALES–BITS AND PIECES FROM TRIATHLON CENTRAL

I had a whole bunch of things rolling around inside my head today. Really not much integration. Kind of like the sport of triathlon right now. But that's okay because sometimes you can't decide to go out for Italian, Mexican or seafood–so you go to a smörgåsbord. And the food tastes great, but you're still a little worried that maybe your stomach and you will end up as the victim of several spices that couldn't reach a compromise.

But you know, sometimes there is no other choice than to throw stuff on the wall and hope it sticks, like I am with the rest of this article.

- Went up to a fellow pro after a race not too long ago and asked him how it went out there. He told me he'd lost then walked away. I thought to myself, "How can you ever lose when you're outside, riding your bike, swimming and running?" Hasn't this guy ever been to a Veterans Hospital or the Special Olympics? I hate ungrateful, crybaby wimps.
- Maybe it's possessive or trivial, but I get really proud when an ex-triathlete does something substantial in another sport. Like Lance Armstrong in cycling or Ray Browning in Nordic skiing. It's just way past cool when somebody you know goes out and nails it in another venue.
- San Diego has been really nice lately. Warm, sunny and chock full of foreign athletes gearing up for the coming season. It doesn't bother me when they come here, just so long as they don't wear their little bikini swimsuits out to the restaurants like they do in Kona.
- Too much complaining in our sport. Entry fees too high. Awards too small. Too hard to get into Ironman. Not enough bagels at the finish line. The same people on the cover of the magazine.
- Hey, who ever said all this shit was supposed to be fair? We could end up like this dude I saw on the side of the road the other day. Only I didn't get a good look at him because he was already inside a black

plastic bag. Kind of puts things in perspective, don't you think?

• Ran into this guy I met awhile back when he came to my house to work on a plumbing problem. He's started running, lost 30 pounds, bought himself a bike, was learning to swim and was as stoked on triathlons as anybody I'd ever seen. He told me he had essentially turned his life around with exercise.

• His name is Ray. He's a real world hero, a nice guy and a damn good plumber. If you live in San Diego and you need a plumber, call him at 270-3179.

• I've never met speed skater Bonnie Blair. But if I was single, I'd ask her to marry me. Sometimes you can just watch the way a person handles themselves in a particular situation and you can tell what kind of person they are. I've met quite a few famous athletes in my travels, but none so honest, uncomplicated, gracious, and unassuming as this speed skater who I don't know from Adam. She and fellow skater Dan Jansen were the class acts of the Winter Olympics.

• I've been thinking about the whole question of equipment lately. Should there be more restrictions, less restrictions, different classes for equipment choices, etc.? And you know what? Life is just too darn short to have some official come up to you in the transition area and disqualify you because your pedal bearings have too light a weight of oil on them.

• The speeches at the awards functions are always too long. Just send our certificates in the mail and with the money you save on trophies, get a decent band to play.

• Some guy came to look at a bicycle I was selling a few years ago. He put on his cleats and went for a test ride. The only problem was that he never came back. Maybe he was poor, or strung out on drugs or something. Heck, I would have given him the bike; it was only worth a few hundred bucks. I was pretty disappointed in humanity that night.

• Scott Molina is sort of unretiring this year. That's good news for a variety of reasons, but mostly because, as one of the only three people in the Desert Lizards Tanning and Triathlon Club, I can go ahead and place that uniform order now.

- I'm really interested in doing a sponsorship deal with Harley Davidson motorcycles. Can someone from Harley please give me a call so we can discuss this? Thanks.
- Race tip #307: During the later stages of an event when you're having trouble concentrating, try to think of the name of your third grade teacher. It'll take your mind off the pain.
- After years of searching for the perfect fluid replacement, I think I've found it: Mix two scoops of vanilla-flavored Endura Optimizer in eight ounces of water. Then add six ounces of French roast coffee and just a pinch of Kahlua. Trust me on this one.

Chapter 4

Triathlon 101

I had a teacher in grade school who constantly reminded us that "learning was fun," and that there was no greater self satisfaction than to see yourself progress to a higher level of skill. Of course, I thought she was nuts. But I was relating her words of wisdom to subjects like spelling, geography and social studies. It didn't occur to me at the time that she was referring astutely to all of life's elements that provide us opportunities for discovery.

My interests at the time were Little League baseball or skateboards, and being able to hit a curve ball or jump a curb didn't strike me as "fun"–it was just something you got better at as you grew up.

Fun, of course, is simply a catch-all word people use to describe activities they enjoy. Many pastimes that would be better described as fulfilling, rewarding, healthy, enlightening or lucrative are pawned off as fun. But that's okay. The term gives a sense of simplicity and naivete in a world that too often tries to be more complicated than it needs to, for no other reason than to scare or intimidate people. Why do you think lawyers have their own language?

To me, triathlon is fun. One of the reasons is the constant advancement it offers. Courses are safer, bikes faster, training methods improved, and so on. Most importantly, I've learned and improved. It would also be safe to say that 90 percent of the people I know in the sport get better every year, regardless of their age.

I don't know if the number is that high in other sports. I doubt it. An illusive psychology of advancement seems to prevail among the demographic population of this sport. Hell, I don't know. Maybe we are all obsessive, compulsive, neurotic, stressed-out yuppies who can't sit still until we perfect everything we do.

Or maybe the subculture of multi-sport enthusiasts understands better than Joe Bag-of-Donuts what my grade school teacher tried to tell us many years ago: learning is fun.

NEW TOYS

One of the unique problems of competing in triathlons during their infancy (mid 70s) was the uncertainty about equipment. Since the number of events worldwide could be counted on ten fingers and ten toes, and the number of people who actually considered themselves triathletes was zero, manufacturers had no interest in or concept of developing a multi-sport product.

How things have changed. Now you can find dozens of companies from small to mega-sized who actively pursue this area by design, development and marketing of cross-training oriented items.

For several years we wrestled with the question of whether to cycle in our running shoes or take the time in transition to put cycling cleats on. Keep in mind that some of those early races had very short bike portions and occasionally more than one bike-to-run or run-to-bike transition.

At one time I tried to modify a pair of running shoes to give them more rigidity on the sole for improved performance while wearing them on the bike. Ultimately the project failed–the specific requirements of each shoe were too contradictory. In addition, the advent of lace locks and velcro closures developed some lightning quick transitions. Ironically, my early drawings resemble some of the cross-training shoes now commercially available.

I'll never forget though, when Mark Montgomery, one of the earliest triathletes, wore his running shoes during the swim of some sort of "micro-length celebrity triathlon." By virtually eliminating any clothing change at all, he easily won the 200 yard swim-two-mile bike-half-mile run affair.

I think we were a fairly creative bunch back then; a bit naive maybe, but the wheels of innovation were always turning. During the pre-

Lycra days, I created a pair of tri-shorts by purchasing a pair of boys-size acrylic stretch warm-up pants and cutting them off at bike short length. They worked great for about three weeks, finally self-destructing in the jacuzzi.

New product designs are often born of necessity, and we needed new equipment to help us facilitate this type of new training and racing endeavor. Nobody had done this kind of thing before, consequently, there were no experts, no precedent, and no "best way to go." Experimentation was the rule.

Along the way, some concepts and designs have stuck and become a necessary piece of equipment, while others never gained popularity. There was a product out several years ago called the TransMaster. I still have one up in the attic that I'm saving for the National Triathlon Museum. It was a type of plastic box platform that you "velcroed" your cycling and running shoes into. This allowed you to slip your feet into the shoes like they were bedroom slippers, step out of the box and go. Not a bad idea, but for a variety of reasons it never really caught on. Can you imagine going to a Bud Light USTS Chicago and seeing 2,000 of these automatic shoe changers in the transition area?

Other products have become almost required equipment. Up until a few years ago you never, I repeat, never, saw guys running in public in bikini-type bathing suits. They have now proven to be the outfit of choice for short-distance races and athletes can be seen parading about the lobbies of headquarter hotels in suits that used to be found only on the French Riviera.

Wetsuits were worn originally for survival in cold water. While the latest suits do indeed provide added flotation, the prevention of hypothermia outweigh any potential inequities. There's just something about being frozen to the core that can only be experienced and not described.

Triathlon has also helped spawn equipment that transcends the sport into other areas. These multi-sport gadgets have helped give credence to the cross-training concept. Clipless bicycle pedals were heavily targeted at the triathlon buyers. Velcro-closure cycling shoes, sleeveless cycling jerseys pockets that double as a running singlet, and aero-type handlebars are all by-products of the triathlon necessities.

Has the advancement in equipment complicated our sport? Has it made it cost-prohibitive to some folks? Sure it has. But it has always been human nature to try and figure out a better way, hasn't it? The automobile engine has certainly caused many problems, but would you rather ride a horse to work every day? (Can you put bike racks on horses?) As for the costs, when technology improves the manufacturing process, products will become cheaper. For example, the first disc wheels were over $3,000. Now you can buy one even better than the originals for under $300.

Ultimately there must be certain constraints that limit equipment advances to reasonable levels. These must not, however, hamper the thought process of those who dream up our next "go fast" gadget. Equipment rules should give us clearly defined, yet loosely restrictive guidelines that manufacturers and athletes and race directors can design, produce and race with.

What is reasonable? The athletes should decide that, not an overbearing governing body. I still can't comprehend how thousands of bike racers can allow a handful of bureaucrats to tell them what color their shorts can be. It's unbelievable! If an athlete wants a new product, is willing to pay a fair price for it and that item is widely available and not unsafe, shouldn't he or she get a shot at it? Or maybe the one with the most toys doesn't always win. You make the decision. It's your sport.

SIGN UP FOR TRIATHLON 101

The first time I heard the word "demographics," I thought it was some kind of sign-painting business. It's a word that people in three-piece suits like to use, kind of like "market share" and "cost-indexing."

Now, I'm no Yale MBA type, but I often tire of the endless triathlon dialogue that permeates most 80-mile bike rides. Sure, disc wheels are nice, but to spend the better part of an hour regaling the technical specifics of each brand gets old. More often than not, when someone in the pack rambles about the top performances at last weekend's triathlon, the great race belongs to the guy who wears the three-piece suit during the week. This is the guy who makes up triathlon "demographics"–mid-to-late 30s, middle-management position in a growth company, goal-oriented, lovely wife, two-to-four kids, drives a Volvo station wagon (with bike racks), earns middle-five-figure annual income, played tennis in the 70s, started running five years ago to lose weight, and is now "Mr. Triathlon."

Obviously the sport attracts all sizes and shapes, but the few studies done on triathlon indicate that a number of individuals, both male and female, have characteristics of the "Yuppie Athlete." (I hate that term.)

Where does all this lead? Personally, I think it's important to know who we are; "We," as in the sport's demographics. Triathlon has been called an "up-scale sport of the 80s"–the fastest growing athletic event in North America and a perfect target market for leisure product corporations. Most of it is probably true. There is no question that marketing types realize that to align your product with triathlon is to access a great deal of discretionary dollars.

But answer me this. What happens when the baby boomers either burn out or drift into another sporting interest? Do their offspring merely step into their shoes? Is triathlon ensconced in today's society to withstand the inevitable tapering off of the growth curve? Both tennis and jogging have survived years of boom and bust. They, of course, had diversity and youth, two areas that triathlon is sorely in need of.

We need to take the sport into the mainstream of our population, not just white collar, suburban, college-educated types. It won't be an easy process. Bikes aren't cheap and pools don't exist in every playground. But the cross-training experience can take a variety of forms; nobody said you had to swim, bike and run to be a multi-sport enthusiast.

The youth are ripe for picking. Certain high school and Ironkid-type programs have laid the foundation, but if the sport wishes any real future, the youth of today need to sign up for Triathlon 101.

THE DOCTOR IS IN

I got sick twice this past winter... so what, you ask. Interestingly, this was double my yearly average for bouts with the bug. They weren't your "simply minor flu symptoms, but I can train through it" illness. This was major germ warfare.

I tried to pass it off to additional exposure through the "kids' play group pipeline", but the truth of the matter is I was simply not as healthy as I should have been. No blaming it on the kid.

How, you ask, can a person not be healthy when he or she trains 40 hours a week, eats well and takes vitamins? Apparently, it's easy. In fact, now that I know what to look for, I can think of several world-class triathletes who aren't very healthy at all. What they are is physically fit. But overall health encompasses so much more; it now appears that training the cardiovascular and musculo-skeletal systems only begins to scratch the surface.

It now appears that such Eastern disciplines as martial arts and Tai Chi that emphasize spiritual and mental training along with the physical are not as far-out as Westerners once thought. Can flexibility be as important as swimming skills? Is percentage of body fat equal to hill-climbing ability? Of course. Everything is inter-related–much more than we realize. We may be able to let one or two less obvious areas of health slip for a while, but in ten days or ten years, it'll catch up and bite us in the ass.

I once knew a guy who was a health freak, left no stone unturned during his quest for physical fitness. Hated the dentist though–almost died from gum disease. Yes, the shin bone definitely is connected to the leg bone. Granted, triathletes are much more overall fit than single-sport specialists, but it's the commitment to physical training that often is the crux of the problem.

Studies have proven that light-to-moderate exercise three times per week will strengthen the immune system. When you get into serious training everyday your ability to avoid bacterial infections and wandering viruses goes down.

Most athletes know that to achieve your potential, you must stress your entire system. Push too hard, go over that fine line, and you become sick or injured. The only real way to discover where that point exists in each of us is to train until we reach the edge, and wait to see what happens.

This is where health and fitness make their true separation. A healthy person is not so concerned with specific athletic performance as he is with how his body performs over the long haul, contributing to quality of life rather than amount of victories.

Interval sessions can be important, but so are good sleeping habits, diet, clean air and a relaxed positive attitude. Mental outlook seems to play a tremendous role in overall health. How many times have you read an article in the tabloids about people who have lived to be well over 100 years old, and had them say that their secret was "proper frame of mind"? Negative people can make you sick, literally. Enough bad vibes can influence the way you feel physically–don't you think?

Is it possible to be a fast triathlete and be healthy at the same time? Sure, but you've got to listen to your body, avoid dumb mistakes, and keep everything in perspective. Here's a starter course:

1. Educate yourself on nutrition and learn to read labels.
2. If you really don't feel like training, maybe your body is telling you something.
3. Vitamin supplements aren't really necessary, but they can be especially helpful if taken the right way.
4. Most countries with a low rate of heart disease advocate a mid-day siesta.
5. If God wanted preservatives in food, He would have put them there.

6. One hundred years from now, who's going to remember who won this year's Ironman? Relax.

7. The sun can make your face look like the dash board of a 1967 Corvair.

8. Drink water until you pee clear once or twice a week.

9. Everything in moderation, except sex, drugs and rock and roll. Those are in the all or none category.

10. Whoever said, "Only the good die young," had a congenital heart problem.

PERTINENT PHRASES–WORDS OF WISDOM TO LIVE BY

I find it particularly impressive when somebody can deliver a grand and purposeful thought in a few short words. When you think about it, most people talk too much anyway. Over the years certain individuals have become known for their ability to fill our minds with human emotions and thought–to be profound without being prolific. Maybe they just said something we wanted to hear or perhaps we were just taken by the moment. Whatever the case, I've tried to gather a few quotes that relate particularly well to the art of athletes.

Here's my collection and interpretation for your visual digestion:

- "Don't bother just to be better than your contemporaries or predecessors. Try to better than yourself." William Faulkner, 1887-1962. In other words, if your primary goal is to beat the guy standing next to you, that's fine. With over one million triathletes worldwide, you've got your work cut out for you. On the other hand, there is only one you.
- "Optimism, said Candide, is a mania for maintaining that all is well when things are going badly." Voltaire, 1694-1778. Remember this one when the starting gun finds you sitting in the Port-O-John.
- "Be careful about reading health books. You might die of a misprint." Mark Twain, 1835-1910. In this day and age, believe none of what you read and only half of what you see. There is a lot of good information on training and racing out there, but none as good as what you learn from experience.
- "In the long run you hit only what you aim at. Therefore, though you should fail immediately, you had better aim at something high." Henry David Thoreau, 1817-1862. This is one of my favorites. We are all going to screw up now and then, right? In the meantime, why not take a flyer? You want to do triathlon? Forget the short crap. Go for the double Ironman.
- "He who would accomplish little must sacrifice little; he who would

achieve much must sacrifice much; he who would attain highly must sacrifice greatly." James Allen, 1864-1912. Unfortunately, you can't do it all. You can do a lot for a while, but sooner or later something gives. You want to be a good triathlete, you have to train. The rewards are there if you work for them.

• "The bow too tensely strung is easily broken." Publilius Syrus, 1st Century B.C. The next time you are on the starting line, relax a bit. Do something to lighten the moment. My favorite is to pee in my wetsuit and let it run down my leg onto someone's toes.

• "A man should never be ashamed to own he has been wrong, which is, but saying, in other words, that he is wiser today than he was yesterday." Alexander Pope, 1688-1744. This, of course, has special significance for those who have competed in the Ironman more than once and fail to learn from year to year that the pain does not go away with experience.

• "People are able to wonder at the height of mountains, and the huge waves of the sea, the vast compass of the ocean, at the circular motion of the stars, and then pass by themselves without wondering at all." St. Augustine, 354-430. Next time you scrape your knee, watch how it heals itself. The human body is an incredible thing. I think we should appreciate the fact and give it more consideration.

• "Looking back, my life seems like one long obstacle race, with me as its chief obstacle." Jack Paar. It's hard to say for sure, but you'd like to believe that there is a tremendous source of untapped potential that lies within each of us. I read the other day that the average person only uses four percent of his mental capacity; pro triathletes use substantially less than that. Let's all go back to college and live in the dorms.

• "When we come to the place where the road and the sky collide, throw me over the edge and let my spirit glide, they told me I was going to have to work for a living, but all I want to do is ride, I don't care where we are going from here, honey, you decide." Jackson Browne, *The Road and The Sky*. I can't touch that one.

WHAT'S YOUR HANDICAP? ADJUSTING RACE TIMES TO PERSONAL BUMMERS

It bothers me when people justify their own inabilities or another individual's successes by chalking it up to genetics. You hear it all the time: "I just wasn't born with the right tools," or "That guy has so much natural talent, he doesn't have to train." Sure, we're all born with different natural abilities and no two people are exactly alike (except maybe for the Puntous twins). But genetic makeup only accounts for some of our successes both on and off the playing field.

Still, I think it's safe to say that some people are born with the tools that–combined with proper training–produce successful athletic performances. Hence, the big question: Should every competitive human endeavor, athletic or otherwise, be accompanied by a handicapping system based upon natural abilities (or lack thereof)?

Of course, we'd have to categorize all competitors according to factors such as age. Children shouldn't compete against adults, and men and women should take separate fields in sports requiring heavy physical contact. But just how far should we take this? Age and sex are acceptable. Should weight be a consideration? How about hometown climate? Or hair color?

Most people agree that when safety and fairness are factors, the decision becomes obvious. But when our natural urge to compete emerges, individual definitions of what is safe and what is fair vary significantly. For example, even though women only make up 10 to 15 percent of an average triathlon field, the prize money is equally divided nine times out of 10. The women who earn that prize money worked just as hard as the men, so it's fair, right? I think so; others don't.

How about the races for women only? They attract more women to the sport. But would it cause a stir if the manufacturers of product aimed at the male market put on an only-for-men race? You answer that one.

The point is, there are no clear lines of demarcation when it comes to categorizing competitors. We all want to compete against people like ourselves without feeling that the guy just in front has an advantage.

Most often, that advantage is merely a perceived advantage. Admit it or not, our successes and failures have less to do with genes than with attitude, preparation, will and other internal forces.

For the sake of fun, though, I thought I would do what the politicians do: determine a handicapping system for triathlon that affects everybody. This isn't based on intangibles; this is real-world stuff, like trying to compete the morning after your kid kept you up all night with the stomach flu or trying to concentrate on winning your age group two days after your spouse wrecked the car.

Factor: You forgot your bike was on the roof rack of your car when you drove into the garage.
Time Adjustment: Subtract four minutes from your finish time. (Relax, we've all done it.)

Factor: You get one of those really painful sores on your, butt just a few days before your first Ironman.
Time Adjustment: Subtract six minutes from your finish time. (Go ahead and do the 112-mile bike ride in your swim suit. It doesn't hurt, trust me.)

Factor: Your girlfriend's father comes to watch you race for the first time. As he waves to you from the spectator area, you realize you're rubbing Vaseline on your private parts in front of him and the 499 people around him.
Time Adjustment: Subtract 30 minutes. (Consider telling him it's for an old war injury.)

Factor: The airline charges you $45 to load your bike, then loses it for two days, bends the rims and says it isn't responsible.

Time Adjustment: Subtract ten minutes. (No. Changing airlines will not help; they're all bad.)

Factor: You get to the transition area and your stuff is covered by somebody else's stuff; this guy decided that your assigned spot was better than his.
Time Adjustment: Subtract five minutes. (Hey, it's war out there.)

Factor: You find (and use) a clean, vacant, port-a-john reserved for VIPs and sponsors.
Time Adjustment: Add two minutes. (Dream on.)

Factor: You eat like a pig to gain seven pounds so you can compete in the Clydesdale division of an upcoming race. At the carbo-loading dinner, as you wolf down your fourth helping of pasta, you hear the race director announce that the Clydesdale division has been dropped from the race this year.
Time Adjustment: Subtract one minute for each pound you gained plus of bonus of five minutes for all the suffering it will take to lose those extra pounds.

Factor: You enter a race called a "freestyle scramble" that's basically a hilly cross-country run along a very narrow trail. There is prize money for first, second and fourth places–but nothing for third place. Near the end of the race, you find yourself in third with a quarter-mile to go. You hide behind a car and let the guy behind you pass so you'll get the fourth-place prize money. Unfortunately, you find out–too late–that the race leader went off the course. So, your little shenanigan puts you back in third place instead of second, where you were before hiding, and fourth, where you thought you were. So, you get nothing for all that trouble.
Time Adjustment: You learn that having a little fun can come back to bite you in the ass every now and then.

P.S. This is a true story. You'll never guess whom it happened to.

STAYING MOTIVATED

The sport of triathlon has changed. Whether you realize it, like it, hate it, appreciate it or simply could care less, nothing you or I can do will make it what it was. Growth is change, unavoidably so. The participants, you and I–whether we are willing to admit it–are not the same people, the same athletes who toed the starting line three, five or 15 years ago. That, too, is a fact of life.

That reality aside, the task at hand is maintaining the same motivation you had the first time you pulled on a swim cap and lined up with 200 other numbered bodies, all milling around nervously in the predawn light, pacing stoically about the transition area, secretly scared shitless–just like you. You had a fire in your belly, fueled by the twin brothers of anticipation and determination. You were psyched.

Over the years, though, the embers cooled, the fuel became scarce and you just plain didn't feel the same way about getting up at 4:30 a.m. to gut your way through another 1.5km S/40km B/10Km R race. But you liked it just the same, you know, the benefits of training and all. Only, the "enthusiasm" had gone down a notch.

You want it back. I want it back. Here's our plan of attack.

1. Ask yourself why you are training, competing, spending $4000 on a bicycle when your car is worth $2000. If you can't come up with a clear reason, keep thinking. This is important. There is no right or wrong reason. Only that you know in your heart why the hell you stay in the sport.

2. Find your origins of passion. Try to think back to what it was that originally attracted you to triathlon. Is your motivation the same? Or, has it changed? Think hard. Write it down. Explore the reasons for a change in thinking. You see, to reach success of a deep personal nature, it is important to love what you do. If you don't truly enjoy the

sport for what it is, move on. Find something you can get fired up about. If you're still in the hunt, but need to make changes in your approach, your "philosophy of triathlon," so to speak, do it with a clear understanding of what it is you need to address.

3. Attack your fears. A poor attitude or loss of motivation can also be disguised as a lack of control or failure to succeed at a given task. I have found that many people fail to reach certain goals because they choose the wrong ones. It is very difficult to attain specific performance goals when there are so many factors beyond our control. For instance, I might say my goal is to win the Ironman again—which is a lofty target. But it is not as simple as just putting down a finishing time or place. If I get terribly fit, win a dozen races, make a lot of people happy and get second in Hawaii, have I failed? It is better to have slightly vague, yet measurable and heartfelt goals that address certain intrinsic rewards, like setting an example for kids, or developing your self-esteem.

If you do what you love and you do it to the best of your ability, the material rewards—money, trophies, even respect your peers—will come naturally.

Some triathletes fear that they will let people down or the pain will become intolerable. Guess again. The truth is, people don't really care how you finish. Your true friends, those whose opinion counts, will only want that you do your best and enjoy your experience.

The pain? Unless you've done something terribly stupid, like going and having a heart attack, you are in control of the pain level. Slow down, it eases; speed up, it gets worse. It really does work that way.

4. Reverse the cycle. If you think you will have a bad race, chances are your prediction will come true. The mind-body connection is tight. You become what you think about and your race is won or lost before the gun goes off. You can reverse this self-fulfilling prophecy by reducing the stress of fear, unrealistic goals and self-doubt and think-

ing positively. Consider that we are all lucky enough to have the opportunity to compete. Life is very short. We must enjoy our endeavors. You don't get another chance.

5. Give something back. You want to get motivated? Find a way to put something back into the sport. Sports psychologist and motivational speaker Manny Edelstein put it this way: "It is in giving that we receive things of real value. Set an example. Be somebody's hero, even if that somebody is you. Believe in what you do so that others can believe in themselves, too." Well said.

When I heard this, I queried Manny further. "How about all the distractions, the politics, the bullshit that takes your eye off of the task at hand?" I asked. He replied, "Those are merely conduits for your inability to focus. If it's not one thing, it would be another. In your mind, to achieve real success, they cannot exist. Ignore the bureaucrats."

WHY IS TRIATHLON DIFFERENT?

What really makes triathlon different from other sports? Sure, it's unique, challenging, different, a bit off-color, but so is field hockey and skeet shooting. But the singular element of this sport that separates it from the pack is the transition–that one spot, that one moment (or so) in time when background and competitive skills are equalized. The situation is obvious and unavoidable–every competitor becomes neither swimmer nor cyclist nor runner, but a triathlete in transition, creating a frantic and frenzied show for family, friends and media to witness.

Yes, the rapid fire "life-in-the-pits" spectacle is purely unique to triathlon. We invented it, we studied it, and we perfected it (ever hear of lace locks back in the 70s?). The transition has been, and remains, the heart and soul of triathlon. It's where competitors return from their bout with the elements (water), struggle to maximize their mastery of technology (two-wheeled transit) and finally confront their own trials and tribulations through the simple and ageless form of physical motion (running).

If you wanted to chronicle the development of the sport through one specific element, a study of transition would be in order. From the early days of "pit-crew assistance" and fresh sock changes to the lightning fast "all-day-in-a-bathing-suit" endeavors of today. The way we move from one sport to the next has reflected the advancements and changes over the years. It has also nurtured the development of a host of products, unknown before triathlon appeared on the scene in the mid 70s. Velcro? What's that? Clipless pedals?

And while the ability to move quickly from one sport to the next has enabled some less-talented athletes to move up in the finish rankings, the stories told from a weekend warrior's experience as he tried to put on someone else's shoes or knocked over a row of bikes like dominoes, is the stuff of legends. We can only hope that as the sport grows and matures, the next generation will recognize the importance of a certain circus atmosphere and maintain the intangible aura of a properly disorganized transition area.

Not too many years ago, people thought that if you were able to hold down a regular job, raise a family and get in two nights a week at the gym, you were a well-rounded individual, a so-called "complete" person.

But the two nights became three, jogging replaced calisthenics, and the word was out that physical fitness improved everything from worker productivity to life span. But that one sport became boring. Soon athletes of all ability levels learned that cross-training was more than a marketing concept to sell more shoes. Triathlon race results were standard fare for cocktail party conversation.

Fast forward to present day 1993 and after two years of a flattened triathlon growth curve domestically, thousands of die-hard, as well as casual triathletes, are looking at one another and saying, "I still dig it, but we need a new rush."

But even though the gluttonous 80s are gone, we can still have our rice cakes and eat it too. Here's how—use triathlon as a stable platform to expand your athletic horizons. The basic axiom of multisport doctrine is that not only is total fitness worth more than the sum of its collective sporting parts, but the process of discovery and adventure is great fun. I'm not advocating an exodus to the latest sports trends (i.e. volleyball, in-line hockey, etc.), but I'm suggesting that like an old marriage, you've got to work at it now and then to keep it interesting.

In the past year I've competed on Nordic skis, paddle boards, in-line skates, mountain bikes and (please don't tell my sponsors) off-road motorcycles. In nearly every case I was at or near the back of the pack. But you know what? I had a great time and not only became a well-rounded sportsman, but a faster triathlete. What more could you want?

MAINTAINING FORM

The comedian Milton Berle once said, "My doctor recently told me that jogging could add years to my life. I think he was right. I feel ten years older already!"

Anybody who has ever experienced the final miles of a hot and nasty triathlon will agree with this. Whether it's a 10K or a marathon, a certain percentage of the field will begin to "lose it" during the latter stages of the run–shedding parts until the final mile looks like one big garage sale. This is no good.

OK, we have all fallen apart before. That's racing. But I can't help, but think that self-implosion is not always necessary. Training factors notwithstanding, a lot of athletes could defer the bonk by concentrating on form and style. Along with form goes speed. If you can maintain your stride length, a relaxed upper body and a general fluid motion, you'll be surprised how your body becomes very efficient with the limited energy you have left.

Take a couple of deep breaths, drop your shoulders, shake out your hands and glide. It may take a little more mental concentration and strength of spirit than you are used to. But, hey, the price of glory isn't cheap.

NAIL IT ON THE BIKE

Cycling is a lot like speaking or listening–we all learn to do it at a very early age, and we never forget how, but few of us really excel at it. Riding a bicycle is a simple activity, really. But to go fast–I mean very fast–requires a whole different mindset. Many of us are inadvertently lulled into a gentle rhythm during the bike leg of a triathlon, satisfied to be out of the water, away from the noisy confusion of a transition area and not yet suffering the muscle-pounding pain of the run. We roll along, take in the scenery and stay out of harm's (and overzealous officials') way. Content to "average" a respectable speed, many of us avoid putting ourselves close to any anaerobic edge for fear of crashing–either on the bike or during the run.

To make your little two-wheeler hum, though, you've got to change your thinking, change the way you approach the cycling leg altogether. A five percent increase in heart rate can often translate into a ten percent increase in speed, which could put you 20 percent higher in the standing. While the rest of the field enjoys the cool wind in their face, you want to put a scowl on yours and attack the bike course. Within reason, let yourself "nail it" a couple of times, just for the hell of it. You'll be surprised how many people you'll pass and that your legs will be no worse off come 10K time. Trust me.

I HEARD IT ON THE GRIPE VINE–MY TRIATHLON LIKES AND DISLIKES

I wonder if *Triathlete* readers might be able to help me out with something. I'm curious, you see, concerning a few things and I don't know how to ask about them without looking foolish or offending someone. You can drop me a short note or whisper in my ear at the swim start when no one is looking.

Anyway, these are my questions:

- How can we convince the female triathletes to keep their fingernails shorter than lethal-weapon length for those free-for-all mass starts?
- Why do some Ironman competitors walk nearly the whole marathon and then sprint the last 100 yards like they are being chased by a saber-toothed tiger? Why not sprint 100 yards somewhere out on the course in the dark, maybe between miles 15 and 16, where there are no spectators? The times would be the same.
- How do some competitors get three flats in one race? do they aim for rocks and glass hoping to put themselves out of the race?
- Why are the German triathletes so good? Did they get the leftover steroids from East Germany or is it because they wear their bikini swimsuits all day long?
- What happened to the 30-hour work week that they told us in 1970 would be the norm by 1990? Forty hours is considered part time, unless you work for the Department of Motor Vehicles.
- How would you feel if you knew you cheated, but didn't get caught? What if you saw your picture on the wall of the post office on the "Drafters" bulletin board?
- What happened to the huge post-race Bud Light parties, $30 entry fees, and the Puntous twins?
- Who stole my bitchin' Yeti mountain bike out of my garage in Boulder?
- What happened to all the 1/2 Ironman distance races?

- What is with the people who train so well, always going very fast, and then get their, butts kicked in the races?
- Who said the I.T.U. guys could appoint themselves king?
- Why don't more races have a short (1 mile) run to get you warmed up and spread out before the bike?
- Why do athletes support races that allow drafting? If someone you despise is having a party, you don't have to go!
- What does everybody do with their race T-shirts when their T-shirt drawer is completely full?
- What a great idea it is to have several big hot tubs at the swim start!
- Why do athletes shave their arms and then swim with a wetsuit?
- When was the last time you wrote a thank you note to a race director?
- Why can't professional baseball players live on a $1 million per year salary? Is their grocery bill higher than ours?
- Why does the alarm go off on race morning just as I finally get to sleep?
- What can we expect from the new crop of pro-triathletes?

While I'm in a "list" mode, here are a few things that leave me in a bad mood:

- When I forget to wash my racing flats that live in the bottom of my bike case for five months a year and they smell like... well, they're really bad.
- When everybody crowds around the posted race results and stares at their splits for an hour.
- Regular trophies with plastic gold figures on top of plastic "wood" bases.
- Airlines that charge $45 for your bike and then crash one of their planes every year.
- Guys who finish in the top five once or twice and act like they're God's gift to the multi-sport world.
- Reporters who ask questions like, "So, what's your favorite event?"
- People who clean their chain with the hotel towels so that next year the

hotel won't allow bikes in the rooms.

And then there are the things I really like about this sport:
- When some girl tells you she named her dog after you.
- Never having trouble falling asleep.
- Having friends in a dozen countries.
- Going to Kona and watching the goofy Ironman parade.
- Eating banana walnut pancakes after a race.
- Being faster than your kids.
- Never having to buy T-shirts or water bottles.
- Hanging out with people who know how to laugh at themselves.
- When a bike shop charges you $20 for a hundred dollars worth of work.

Remember, the only stupid question is the one that is never asked.

Chapter 5

What Is It You Do Again?

Every year when I fill out my event form for the Ironman, I come across the section that asks you to state your chosen profession. Each year, I write down what I then consider myself to be, yet without fail the person reading the application ignores my designation and types in "Professional Athlete." Why is that? Why can't they believe I am a sportsman, or clothing manufacturer, or writer, or teacher, or even the grossly generic "entrepreneur"? They certainly believe Paul Huddle when he claims he is a Lambach Instructor, or Tom Gallagher when he lists his occupation as Crossing Guard.

Why do I have to be considered simply a professional triathlete? You see, I've always wrestled with that label. It's almost an oxymoron– *professional* denoting "for profit" and *triathlete* giving an image of multiple activities in pursuit of pleasure. Yet it does work, and for some people, work well.

But in the early days of the sport, I had a hard time explaining to those who asked that I earned a living, and a nice one at that, by swimming, cycling and running. Maybe it was the fact that I was always involved in many aspects of sport and had parallel interests, professionally speaking. Or maybe I just couldn't believe I was living out the boyhood fantasy of making "the show," or earning bucks to play a game of sorts.

In the last twelve years, I have tried to understand where my space was, who my peers were, and just what the hell I was supposed to do.

I was one of the first triathletes. There were no role models, no older guys in whose footsteps to follow. Everything was uncharted territory, and I liked it that way. Besides, the idea of being "typical and normal" always bored me stiff.

And so we continue to evolve as a collection of sporting enthusiasts, sometimes forced by our individuality, and sometimes inspired by others' personal acts of valor and courage. Always happiest, though, when we make our own decisions to press on and become more whole because of it.

Yes, I am stoked to do this job. It is, as they say, good work if you can get it. And I am proud of my accomplishments, though in a way that you might not expect. The victories are not "icing on the cake" or even "a piece of the puzzle." They are simply a partial result of some greater process–or maybe just of going to work each day and getting the job done.

JUST A FAD?

I am constantly amazed by fads and why certain things become "in" while others are booted out as quickly as they're created. Who decides what's hip and what's not, anyway? Is it manufacturers and advertisers of products who decide what we're supposed to be doing and wearing in pursuit of created markets for their goodies? Could such classics as the Frisbee and mini-skirt be simple creations of the capitalist system? Personally, I shudder to think that my treasured skateboard was created for anything, but unadulterated fun.

Maybe fads are merely the reflection of a society that has become so shallow and hedonistic that it must constantly search for new and different forms of pleasure; heck, I dunno. Variety really is the spice of life, but if your efforts to follow fashion are merely the result of a desire to be doing or saying the accepted thing, then something is wrong. Being cool is a basic human need; trying to be cool and getting caught at it, and you're a nerd, a fred, a dwid... get outta town!

Take the much-maligned state of California, a veritable spawning ground for innovation. While the rest of the country makes fun of our sprout-eating drivers of convertibles on the way to sessions with the psychiatrist, guru or personal-fitness consultant, the world emulates the state's every outdoor move. California didn't invent surfing, jogging or aerobics, but it wasn't until after residents of the state embraced those activities that they went mainstream and became fads or trends.

It's been the same with the triathlon. One reason I think that so many fads start here is because there's an open attitude, and people will try anything once. If it's worth a darn they'll keep doing it and someone else will give it a try. A fad is born. I'm kind of answering my own question here about where fads come from; advertisers and manufacturers can help create fads, but I think there has to be something of real value to begin with.

So, are triathlons a fad? You bet! Many people have joined the sport's ranks because it's an "in" thing to do. The big question, however, is whether the sport is more than a fad; will it have some staying power? Or will it pass as quickly as it came? I don't think so.

First of all, the type of person attracted to the sport is generally not overly concerned with fad or fashion. I mean, have you ever seen a blow-dryer in the transition area? Secondly and most importantly, the sport demands a real commitment; you can't just go out and buy something and become part of the trend. You've got to buy stuff and train your butt off.

It demands more commitments than marathons even, and marathoners were thought to be pretty committed people. You can go out and buy a pair of shoes, train for a few months and do your marathon. But triathlons demand lots of equipment and the attainment of three skills: swimming, biking and running. It's real work becoming a triathlete, and once you've done all that stuff for your first race, it just isn't natural to bag it without doing more races.

So welcome new triathletes to our ranks and make it easy on them if you can.

Yeah, triathlons are kind of like a hip fad, and many people are attracted to the sport for that reason. But don't look down on them for it, because to get in on this show, you have to really pay your dues. It's the same with the sport itself. Passing fad? No way. Not when you have hundreds of thousands of people training for months and spending millions of dollars on equipment to be involved in this sport. They're in the sport for the long haul and the sport's here for the long haul. The sport demands more commitment than any regular fad, and the triathlete has to put out in a way that superficial trend followers can't hack.

UNDERGROUND CULT RACES

When I was in grade school back in the 60s, one of the most controversial topics was the teaching of what was called "new math." I don't think I fully understood what was so new about it. After all, who of us sitting in those cramped wooden school desks was so adept at the manipulation of numbers that a slight change in the way it was taught to children could be so monumental? Certainly not I.

The mental process and challenge of working with figures was indeed appealing. But somewhere along the way it appeared to me that math got complicated purely for the sake of complication; sort of like the teachers had to justify their jobs or something. I'm sure that calculus and trigonometry have applications to science in many ways and that the process of enabling X to equal Y contributed to the cure of some dreaded disease. But every once in a while I long for simplicity in numbers and simplicity in life.

Learning the multiplication tables reminds me of the earliest triathlons–not that I learned those skills concurrently. As I remember, there were very few triathlons in 1962.

But as the sport grows and more people become involved, some of the innocence wears off. Things change. Simplicity gives way to computerized registration. Camaraderie takes a back seat to sponsor exposure. Sometimes growth is not a bad thing, especially if you can gracefully surrender the things of youth. Growth provides opportunities for thousands of people to have a triple-sport experience. It would be selfish to say, "Hey, we like it just the way it is–the class is full."

With an increase in numbers comes an increase in complexity–a necessity if a race with 2,000 entrants is going to be safe and well-organized. Without things like draft marshals and transition area security, you'd have chaos.

In these rapidly changing times, it's refreshing when you can slip back a few years and find what is affectionately known as an underground cult race (UCR). Kind of like balancing your checkbook without a calculator. For an event to be labeled a UCR, several rules apply. First, no advertising of any sort is allowed to publicize the event. Word of mouth is all that is necessary. Second, no money is involved. No entry fee, no prize money. UCRs never obtain permits, most are held on dirt roads and trails and most importantly, if anybody gets hurt, no one is legally responsible. People simply disappear, obviously afraid of race director's enemy number one—the "I screwed up so I'll sue somebody" syndrome.

There are several classic underground cult races in San Diego each year, races that I await with a passion. An unwritten code prevents me discussing the times and places of these events, but they are put on by long-time locals, people more interested in preserving the tradition of backyard events, and not the search for "big bucks."

Some of these races have a theme, others are made unique by the terrain or the personality of the race director. The competition is usually fierce—bragging rights for a year are highly desirable, but the fun quotient is always the priority.

UCRs' enemies are hidden inside progress. Residential housing threatens running trails. New wilderness laws prohibit mountain bikes in some areas. And everywhere cities fear the dreaded deep-pocket lawsuit. Tradition is important, though, and everywhere there are people who remember their past and wish to preserve just a piece of it—whether it be their first experience with the "new math" or funky little race they always enjoyed to the max.

UCRs exist in every city. Some of them cross the line and do a bit of advertising, charge an entry fee and submit to the pressures of growth. How can you deny hundreds of people who want to partake? The challenge is to keep the flavor. A few have managed to exist in both worlds—the Tug's Tavern Swim-Run-Swim, for example, is one of the oldest biathlons in the country and arguably the most colorful. Others have gone full high-tech with a noticeable change in atmosphere.

There's no doubt that the future will invariably bring a change to the type of events that we have to choose from–especially in major metropolitan areas.

But wouldn't it be nice to be able to get together one Sunday in February each year to race up the side of a local mountain for the 15th-annual, underground run to the top?

HAVE YOU EVER WONDERED WHY...?

I don't recall the event, but some years ago I raced in a triathlon that required the competitors to have their numbers marked on them the night before the race. At the time this struck me as odd, even comical. What were these athletes supposed to do–not take a shower? And how about the numbers rubbing off onto the bed sheets. How would you like to have 389X stenciled on your pillow for life?

But on second thought, the race director must have been a genius, way ahead of his time. There was a recent proposal to require all triathletes to have their social security numbers permanently tattooed onto their arms, so as to avoid long lines of pre-race body marking. What a great concept! I hope they let us do them in neon colors.

Anyway, I particularly like these old scenarios. They provide a tremendous opportunity to learn why we do the things we do. Sometimes, it takes a little probing, but there's usually a lesson or two hidden in the strangeness.

Most of what I know about triathlon, I learned in the first race I entered. Sure, you learn more about the sport and most importantly, more about yourself, each time you toe the starting line, but who can ever forget the first anything? I have vivid memories of my first wave, the first time I heard the word Vietnam, driving a car all alone and my first bike crash. Not that there's any relevance here, but think about the first time you entered the water with dozens or even hundreds of other humans, all kicking and splashing and trying to swim around an over-sized balloon. It may all seem silly to you now, but at the time, you had more butterflies than a field of lilies.

And when you got off the bike to run you suddenly had great respect for those who had so bravely gone before you. You finally experienced the "Kona Shuffle" in all its glory.

When it was all over you were stoked and you learned the same things we all did our very first race:

- There are few things as rewarding as setting a goal, working towards it and achieving it. Period.
- Luck is where preparation meets opportunity.
- Time (and success) wait for no one, especially those who blow dry their hair in the transition area.
- The amount of encouragement you receive is equal to the amount you offer (see Golden Rule).
- People who draft probably don't lift the toilet seat when they go number one.
- Having good equipment is like starting the game on the 30-yard line. Getting it for free is like having someone run the ball into the end zone for you.
- If you race merely for the tributes from others, you will be at the mercy of their expectations.
- The pain in your legs and lungs will go away in a few hours. The pain in your heart from a failed attempt at finishing may take a little longer.
- Laughter and a cold beer will cure most of the aches and pains.

So there you have it. Most of what you need to know to achieve personal success in triathlons you learned the very first time you crossed the finish line. You just didn't realize it. I certainly didn't. And now, 14 years and some 200 races later, the lessons still come, but are much more vague and not always in black and white. The issues are heavier, the consequences higher. The grays and half-tones often cloud what's right and wrong. I have a list though.

A list of things I desperately want to know before I clean out my locker:

- Why don't race directors mark the course with huge chalk arrows three days before the race so athletes can practice it?
- Why doesn't the Ironman ever have course mile markers?
- Why do some athletes get chain grease all over the carpet in hotel

rooms? Do they do this at home?

• Why has Tri-Fed come down like a load of bricks on the use of illegal drugs (which hasn't been a big problem yet) and yet they still allow lead riders to motor-pace behind media vehicles at dozens of races?

• Why aren't there more kids and women in triathlons?

• Why do the airlines charge $30 to ship your bike when you only have one other small bag?

• Why do they always give away T-shirts? How about beer mugs or paper-weights or something?

• When will race directors and volunteers get the respect they deserve?

• When will the girls realize that Kenny Souza should not be a sex symbol?

TRANSLATING "TRIATHLONESE"

The sport of triathlon attracted some rare individuals in its early days–men and women who were different from the norm. There were guys who only shaved on alternate Thursdays and wouldn't dream of wearing neon shorts, unless of course they became an unpopular choice. What sticks in my mind the most are the quotes in early articles about the sport. Obviously, very few people were worried about image or sponsors. They called it like they saw it: good, bad or ugly.

With so many walks of life now filling the ranks of entrants, the triathlon certainly attracts a wide variety of people; some verbal and outgoing, others quiet and introspective. Whatever the case, I find it amusing and sometimes annoying when the visible people, or any competitor for that matter, says one thing, but really means another.

With that in mind I've put together a brief translation guide that will help get the real message out without spending too much time wading through the garbage:

- When a semi-talented age group athlete decides to race pro, he or she says, "I just want to train hard for a couple of years and see what I can do." They really mean, "this is a great excuse to be a bum and take some time off from work."
- When a course is described as, "challenging, with undulating terrain" you might as well bring along a 24-tooth freewheel because it's probably a killer.
- When your best friend (and arch-rival in training) comes up to you after the race, (in which he beats you) and says "if the race would have been another mile you would have caught me," he really means "if the race would have been another mile, I would have beaten you even worse."
- When you see a new product advertised in the magazines that says "guaranteed to take minutes off finish time," what it really should say is "guaranteed to take minutes off of my finish time, because if you

buy it, I make more money and have to work less, so I get to train more."

- When the race application says "a rustic course, with typically metropolitan roads through a scenic downtown area," it means you don't want to be on the course after dark. Consider offering to pace your Marine buddy.

- When the carbo dinner is advertised as "pasta-pasta-and-more-pasta," don't expect a quiet, relaxing pre-race meal. In fact, you'll probably be lucky to get any sauce.

- When the airlines say "due to weight restrictions, your bike was delayed until the following flight," they really mean, "one of our baggage handlers screwed up and forgot to carry the bike out to the plane."

- When your boss says to you, "I really don't think you are focused enough on your job at the moment, maybe you're exercising too much," he really means, "If I wasn't so overweight and stressed out, I'd get in shape and kick your, butt in them there triathlons."

Actually, there a few things that go just the other direction–understatements if you will.

- As hard as anyone says the course can be at the Bud Light Ironman in Hawaii, it's worse. Much worse. People have short memories. The past few years in Kona have yielded near ideal conditions. It'll be different this year. Expect the winds from hell and be pleasantly surprised with mild, 20 knot headwinds.

- Scott Molina is very understated. Most people will tell you they rode 50 miles today when they probably went 38. If Molina says he had a "pretty tough week," you can assume it would put most people in the hospital. He's a nice balance in a sometimes artificially inflated world. Then again, deadmen tell no lies.

- All in all, the truth seems to be much easier to find in our sport than it does in the corporate sector. But then, I don't know; I've never really spent time there. Or have I?

WELCOME TO TRIATHLON–WHAT A BEGINNING TRIATHLETE SHOULD KNOW

As the sport of triathlon continues its maturation process (you know, growing up), the initial excitement of its honeymoon period begins to wane. More people do get involved each year, swelling the ranks and filling the chairs at the omnipresent "carbo-loading party." But not at the same levels as experienced during the boom period of the late 80s.

With that in mind, I have decided that it is the responsibility of the existing constituency to begin an aggressive campaign to enlist new members into our fold. And since part of the problem with any new experience for people is lack of background knowledge, I have begun to compile a "Welcome to Triathlon" primer. Listed below are excerpts from the initial draft. Any comments or suggestions?

Who's Who
There is often a need to know just who the players in a triathlon are:

- If an athlete is wearing his swimsuit everywhere, including out to dinner, the hotel lobby and the awards ceremony, he is unmistakably a German.
- If you notice an athlete sitting in the corner reading a large, technical-looking book, he or she is not a triathlete.
- When you notice that a person is still wearing his or her numbers on their arms and legs the day after the race, this will indicate a first-timer who will be more than happy to share the experience with you.
- If you spot a man running a race and he is wearing cutoff Levi's and black socks, you are probably not eyeing the race leader. (If you do see a race leader wearing cutoff Levi's and black socks, you are in Kansas, Dorothy. See "Location Finder" below.)
- When you see the lead woman and she has long hair and a tight bikini, make sure there are no tattoos: You may actually be watching Kenny Souza.

• If you see an older gentleman wearing a navy blue blazer who is having an intense conversation with someone who looks oddly similar to him (and neither one is watching the race), try to be friendly toward them. They are either Tri-Fed officials, race sponsors, the hotel management or the father of the young girl you were checking out–none of whom you can afford as an enemy.

• A man surrounded by 200 Australian triathletes is usually a bartender.

Location Finder

One of the interesting aspects of triathlon is that many of its followers travel a fair bit to race and "make the scene." Study these points before you get on board.

• As the plane begins to descend, and out of the window you behold the most bleak and barren piece of real estate you have ever seen, you are either arriving for the first annual Lunar Landing Triathlon, or you are simply back in Kona.

• When a baggage handler says, "Sorry, mate, your push bike didn't make the flight. Fair dinkum, maybe tomorrow," then sees you are getting worried, grins broadly and pulls your bike out from behind a door, you must be in Australia.

• When the race director picks you up in a big ole Chevy truck and says, "I hope y'all like it hot," you are most likely somewhere south of the Mason-Dixon Line. (Caution: Don't wear your lime-green tights out to the rib joint restaurant.)

• When someone invites you along to run with a few friends on a Tuesday morning and you arrive to what looks like the start of a major 10K, you are in San Diego. It has to be San Diego, because in any other city you'd be arrested for staging a parade without a permit.

Triathlon Nuances

Every sport has its particulars that create a unique atmosphere and identity. These should help you get a handle on triathlon's singular details:

• If you are anxious to meet a professional triathlete, look for someone with chrome sunglasses, no body hair, and lots of sponsors' logos plastered across his or her clothes. Tell the person that you will sponsor him or her, and you have a friend for life.

- If you are interested in learning about a triathlete's nutritional habits, go to the library and check out The True Story Behind the Smorgasbord.

- If you would like to see where a triathlete lives, drive around until you see a garage that houses a 1972 Volkswagen Squareback, three racing bikes, a plethora of old running shoes, a poster of Mark Allen with horns and a goatee drawn on his face and a half dozen empty Bud Light cans on the workbench.

MULTISPORT MUSINGS–WHAT WOULD IT BE LIKE IF I HAD MADE FIRST STRING IN HIGH SCHOOL FOOTBALL?

Here's my 1993 collection of rhetorical questions, at least as they pertain to sports.

What would it be like if:

• Boxing promoter Don King was the executive director of Tri-Fed?

• Dave Scott tried out for chess instead of swimming in high school?

• Drafting violations carried a monetary penalty?

• You could get bonus points for swimming, butterfly throughout the entire swim segment?

• The guys who invented triathlons had ridden motorcycles instead of bicycles?

• Awards ceremonies started on time? (Would that mean I'd be late?)

• You could go to college on a triathlon scholarship?

• Races were not allowed to start before nine o'clock in the morning?

• Political disputes could be won or lost by a team time trial?

• The Ironman was held in Antarctica?

Don't you think that...?

• We should all boycott airlines that rip us off for $45 bike transportation charges?

• We should volunteer to pay an extra 75 cents each to the race organizer if he or she would get a really good band for the awards ceremony?

• It's a crime that there aren't more triathlons for kids, women, and guys over 35 years of age?

• Guys who complain about all the things that are wrong with triathlon should be given positions on Tri-Fed's Board of Directors?

• Most triathlons on TV are about as interesting as a telethon?

• There should be more TV races anyway?

• There are few things that taste as good as an ice cold Bud Light at the finish line under a tall, shady tree?

Triathlon truisms:
• The more you spend on a bike, the faster it goes.
• The better you look in a race, the faster your bike goes.
• If we believe everything we hear about triathlon in the Olympics, I'd already have two gold medals on my mantle.
• We all started near the back of the pack, and sooner or later, we'll all end up near there.
• The more you give back to the sport, the more you'll receive.
• If you really want a good press agent, hire your grandmother.
• If the application says "flat and fast" don't buy any real estate from the race director.

You're not really a triathlete unless:
• Your coworkers complain of the chlorine smell around your desk.
• You have a scar on your left hip from more than one bike crash.
• You refuse to throw away your first pair of Tinley running shorts.
• You schedule meetings with your boss around noon swim training.
• There are three pairs of goggles in the glove box of your car.
• You're willing to accept a transfer at work–to San Diego or Boulder.
• Your spouse, who used to hassle you about all that training, now swims two lanes down from you–with the fast group!
• You've spent enough money on entry fees to send your kid through college on the five-year plan.
• Each year, when the ideas of March bring tax time, you scheme for hours trying to write off all those training and travel expenses.

Ten tips for sparking your enthusiasm for triathlon:
• Go watch a baseball game and check out the beer belly on the left fielder.
• Take a vacation to one of those exotic races you've read about in mag-

azines, like Chile, Nice or Japan.

• Start a triathlon club and vote yourself president and athlete of the month. (The long-term strategy for triathlon tax write-offs.)

• Supplement your training with a new and different sport, like nordic skiing, rollerblading, snow shoeing or mountain biking. Make sure it's an activity that allows you to show off your quads, though.

• Give a friend an entry into a race for a present (then write it off as charity).

• Stop for a moment and consider how lucky you are to have two good legs, two good arms and a heart that works like a Mercedes-Benz.

What would you do if:

• A cigarette company sponsored a major triathlon?

• You could win a gold medal in the Olympics, but only live another ten years?

• You were sprinting down Alii Drive in Kailua-Kona to win the Gatorade Ironman, with thunderous applause from fans lining both sides of the street, only to realize your shorts had fallen down to your knees? (And all along you thought that feeling in your legs was lactic acid buildup.)

• A shaggy looking kid appears at your door for a date with your 16yearold daughter, and you notice he drives an old van with soiled curtains and a cot instead of seats, but he's wearing an Ironman finisher's T-shirt?

• You were disqualified from a race you weren't even attending because your buddy borrowed your race bib (and maybe your credit card)?

• Discovered, after doing a season's worth of intervals at the local elementary school track, that the track was 40 yards shy of a standard 440? (No wonder your quarters were so impressive!) I'd keep it quiet and keep going to that track.

• You suddenly realized that life just isn't that long and you better get out there and enjoy that 60mile ride with your wife?

FITTING LIFE INTO TRIATHLON

I didn't get into exercise at a young age. It got into me. Just as a friend who comes to stay with you becomes a part of your life and ends up moving in, athletic training just showed up on my doorstep one day and moved in.

It took more and more of my days, gradually displacing other interests that I had put on the back burner. Training was my school; racing was my test. I was filled with excitement as my lifestyle evolved from the nine-to-five regime into one of play for profit. It was hard, with few guarantees, but I knew that what I had lacked in ability, I would make up for in work ethic.

Then five years passed, and I had a daughter. Training for triathlons was no longer the No. 1 priority in my life anymore. Four more years, another child, a variety of business commitments, and long gone were the days when I could relax between workouts.

But to "make it" in this world, you have to adapt to change, not force it. Some things cannot be controlled. The harder you push, the harder it pulls. So it goes with the integration of family and fitness. Both are important, and both can be attained through a complicated system of checks, balances, prioritizing and disguise. There are rules to follow, though, and sacrifices must be made.

If you see a man or woman standing on the victory stand, and you know they have a family, he/she either: a) has no social life; b) is a "trust-funder"; c) has a very understanding spouse; d) lies about how good a parent he/she is; or e) all of the above.

Fortunately, one of the things we have some control over is the timing and size of the family that we choose to create. Even though I was married at a young age (for my generation), the trend is for people to wait now, and let their careers become established. This also delays

the commitment of rearing children until, on average, the early 30s–
the time when most people realize several things about their bodies:
1. They can't fit into their cheerleader outfits.
2. Playing touch football with the guys creates more aches and pains
than it did in college.
3. It really is hard to find a scale that doesn't lie.

So, when you come home, you find your wife reading Parenting magazine. It seems that everything happens at once: the job promotion that
necessitates a couple of late nights a week, the need to lose the spare
tire on your waist and the cute little guy in the nursery window that
has your eyes. They told us college would be more fun than high
school, and the work force more interesting than college–just get into
your 30s, and you can begin to enjoy life. Yeah, right.

We make our bed, though, and we lie in it. Having a passel of young
ones and thinking you're going to be able to sneak in a nap on Sunday
afternoon, let alone a three-hour bike ride, is pure fantasy. Unless, of
course, you call yourself a professional. Then you can train whenever
you want. Now the IRS has strict rules about being a "professional" at
anything. But your relatives don't know that, and as long as you can
justify it in your own mind, you're okay. Until little Bobbie comes up
to you and says, "Hey, Dad, I thought you said we could play catch
today." Well, I don't know about you, but I'm a sucker for those
puppy-dog eyes and a well-oiled mitt.

These kind of decisions have to be made all the time, and believe me,
they get harder as that spare tire gets bigger. So what do you do? Simple. You do what every self-respecting, over-worked, stressed-out,
modern parent does–you schedule your day down to the minute: 20
minutes for Kathy's dentist appointment, 32 minutes to make dinner,
19 minutes on the NordicTrack, and so on.

Heaven forbid someone should hold you up, because if you have to
take something out, it's the workout that gets the boot. That's why
your boss, or the doctor or even the policeman directing traffic feels

your wrath when you miss your 41 minute run. It's always their fault you were late and got behind. If this happens a lot, you simply move your training up the priority list until it receives the attention it deserves. This, of course, is a personal decision that must take into account a variety of factors.

During the birth of our first child, when my wife was in the early stages of labor the doctor assured me that nothing would happen until well into the day and she would be watched carefully by a staff of competent nurses. Could I sneak out for a short run around the hospital grounds? Of course, said my wife. Was I going over the edge on this one? Absolutely. (Remember what I said about being a professional and justifying anything in your own mind?)

So you organize and you prioritize; you try and do everything; make everybody, including yourself, happy. And sooner or later, something goes bump in the night. Your boy is sick, your plane delayed, your company moves you to Mississippi and the teenage baby-sitter starts to call you by your first name. Things have to change.

You find that one copy of *Parenting* and see a photo of a parent jogging with her kid in one of those ultra-cool three-wheeled strollers. Therein lies the answer. Take the little dudes–no, take everybody with you. The spouse, the dog, the in-laws, you name it–they're going to work out. This requires a fair bit of planning and coordination, but trust me, in the long run, it's the only answer. Sometimes the Tinleys show up at the park with a van full of toys, kids, pets, and sundry items needed to keep everybody happy while Dad can do a few intervals on the grass before taking the helm as Mom sneaks in a little run.

Once you've perfected this concept of killing six birds with one stone, you're ready for the ultimate in family/training integration–the "I'll ride the bike and meet you guys in the next town" vacation. Happy trails!

Chapter 6

The Road Less Trampled

If any man seeks for greatness, forget greatness and ask for truth and he'll find both.
Horace Mann, 1796-1859

The late, great running doctor and author George Sheehan was a philosopher of sorts. His words, both written and spoken, offered his followers a unique, insightful perspective on life's daily occurrences.

Reading some of George's works, once or twice I have forgotten that the piece was a magazine article intended for the consumption of thousands and not a personal letter to me.

Years later I would reflect, often in my own writings, about the style and method of some other writer's piece that explored not the *how* of this crazy sport, but the *why*. And though the message and quality varied, the common theme was the search for truth. Though often amateurish in effect, the process was clearly self-cleansing; like the way you feel after writing a long letter to an old friend, spilling your guts on issues you wouldn't usually approach with a cocktail or three.

If you consider it, we all have our own methods of finding what's real, of weeding through the bullshit and making sense of this hectic, mixed-up and often confused society we live in. Heaven knows it's not easy to understand the meaning and beauty of this world when you're stuck in 5:00 o'clock traffic and some asshole just rear-ended you. But as athlete's, we have a distinct advantage. Not only is exercise a wonderful way to relieve the stress upon too many white mice in the box, it is also a perfect vehicle by which to travel to a more sane location no matter where you are.

I remember the first time I went to Tokyo and felt completely overwhelmed by the oppressive crowds and manic pace of the city. After a 90 minute jog through a large park, the oppression became excitement, and the pace–opportunity. In other words, it's attitude–plain and simple. You know, the half-full, half-empty sort of thing.

We all have the ability to let that optimism flow. It's just that some people have let life's negatives stomp it right out of them. I honestly don't believe that serial killers are born that way. They may have a propensity for violence, but it's the ugly shit they haven't overcome along the way that puts them over the edge.

You just have to find your own release valve so that when the tension inside gets too high, you just open the valve and balance the pressure.

IS TIME ON MY SIDE?

Think about this. If you waste just 30 minutes a day for one year (which is easy to do), at the end of the year you'll have pissed away 180 hours, or the average waking time of eleven whole days.

Think about this. If you ran for one hour each day for 40 years, you will probably add several years to your life, not to mention improving the general quality of it. If you took that hour and saved it, you'd have two complete years, negated of course by the stress that wasn't released by a daily run.

The study of time is fascinating to me. Consider the fact that during our lifetime we will spend an estimated six months sitting at stoplights, eight months opening mail, and two years attempting to return phone calls. These kind of statistics are no doubt developed by some kind of priority management consulting company who wants your business, but nevertheless, if they are half true, they are shocking. What they don't consider is the quality of time. Maybe two years of phone calls was something most enjoyable to you. In a day and age of fast-pace living, where the invention of another time-saving device is worth a guaranteed million, it's probably time to look harder at how we spend our precious free time instead of constantly trying to save, prioritize, and maximize it.

Time and its relation to athletics takes a unique twist. Sporting contests are usually against another person, yet the element of time is often a factor. How much time is left? Did I break my best time? Is his time under the record? I can't last another minute! Doesn't it seem ironic to you that countless people spend time exercising in order to hold back the inevitable process of aging? It shouldn't; when people are fit, their quality of life is improved.

People like to associate athletic performances with times. It gives them a standard by which to compare themselves to others. Trying to rate the quality of one's experience during a race to that of another competitors is difficult. There is no trophy for reaching the "highest level of harmony with oneself." Maybe there should be. No, that would go against the idea of competing for such intrinsic awards as self-satisfaction, personal growth and confidence. You can find athletes who will quote you his or her mile splits for the past five years of races. It's a little harder to find someone who might say, "Yeah, at mile 22 of the 1984 Boston Marathon, I reached a level of tranquility that only rivals my first self-discovery at the 1982 Pike's Peak race."

People tend to focus more on the use of such things as money and material possessions, which are renewable, than they do about the use of their time, which is irreplaceable. And as athletes, we often get caught up in the "more is better" syndrome. If 100 miles per week on the bike is good, then 200 is twice as good. If we enjoyed competing in three triathlons this summer, won't six or seven be better next year? This, of course is a great falsehood.

I've always envied people who know how to say no, who can delegate without feeling guilty, who aren't a slave to minor details. It takes a certain mastery of one's athletic career to be confident in one's training and racing program and to be satisfied with a performance, regardless of the rankings against a competitor. And of course, common sense suggests there is an important difference between knowing what to do and actually doing it.

Triathlon has experienced a meteoric rise in popularity in recent years. As triathletes, we are great consumers–entering every race we could find, buying all the latest gear and devouring each item of information on training, racing and gossip, as if our careers depended on it. (In some case it did!) Things are changing now. While growth is constant, races may not double in size each year. It's probably time to evaluate our own place in the sport. Ask why and how to get where you're going–wherever it is. Enjoy the experience. As competitors, most of us only have another 50 or so years. It's really not that long a time.

IRONMAGIC

There are varying opinions as to what competition is, or what it should be. For some, it's the struggle to climb the perennial corporate ladder to beat out the guy in the next office–a career-long race to achieve what the sociologists call "Upward Mobility." In this arena, the "carrot" is more money and more power. It doesn't really matter. They have become interchangeable.

For some, competition is reduced to a daily struggle to feed and house their family, put a little away for tomorrow and to strive for a bit of happiness through it all.

But for a small cross-section of others, competition takes on a different meaning. Their concept of battle can be considered loftier than, say, the struggle for legal tender. It can also be considered petty and self-focusing when compared to the wars of survival that go on daily in back streets of cities around the world.

Whatever the opinion, those who seek to compete in sports do so because they have a specific need to be met. Somewhere there is a hole that needs to be filled. Their involvement in a race, game, or match, gives them the arena in which to seek their goal. Therein lies the secret.

For years, race directors, promoters, television producers and corporate heads have tried to reproduce the magic that is Ironman. Some have come close. There are better organized races. There are safer races. There are more beautiful courses and there are, no doubt, much easier triathlons of the same distances.

But none have been able to reproduce the feeling that one gets from Kona. It's not that the event is flawless. It is not. It's not the fact that it's a World Championship and that entry is limited to a fraction of those who really want to race. It's not TV. It's not even the fabled aloha spirit that thousands of local volunteers graciously bestow upon the competitors.

The magic of Ironman is a perplexing, baffling and seemingly inexplicable desire in the hearts and minds of its competitors, both real and imagined. When men and women hear about the event, it strikes a chord, waking a sometimes dormant primal instinct to do battle. War, however, has become quite unpopular in the last century. But the innate need to challenge oneself, to explore one's physical and mental limits, has remained an integral part of the human experience of many.

For the multitudes plodding along in the middle and upper socio-economic classes, life has indeed become relatively easy since 1950. Even the turbulent 60s, where self-expression was the rage, produced so many "conveniences" that even the personal conflicts of Southeast Asia eventually gave way to a station wagon in the suburbs. By the end of the 70s, my peer group needed a cause. Not political, not environmental, but a personal Roman colosseum in which to pass the rites of manhood–without getting arrested.

By no means of the imagination am I trying to raise the Ironman to global proportions. Far from it. One day, one sporting event. No more, no less. There is a reason for the magic though, a correlation between an individual's hunger for personal triumph and John Collins' challenge to a handful of Honolulu athletes.

Ironman was the first. Like a first love, it's not easily forgotten. My fondest memories are not of running down Alii Drive with victory in hand, but of the unexpected and innocent third place my first time on the Queen "K" Highway.

Ironman has given me and thousands of other competitors opportunities–chances to experience a multitude of human feelings in a few short hours. And while those feelings were at least 50 percent painful, in the end, I know that I, as well as others, have become better people because of it. For that, I am grateful.

Could something else have provided me the same forum for personal growth? Probably. It could have been another triathlon, maybe another sport–hell, we could have all been taken by a religious cult. But we weren't. And Ironman lives on.

For a growing subculture of endurance enthusiasts, it remains the Holy Grail, one of the last bastions of elite world-class sporting events that reserves a spot or two for "everyman."

That too, will most likely change, the lottery being a victim of the event's own evolution. The event can no longer exist in a vacuum, sculpting its own set of standards, seemingly detached from the rest of the triathlon world. It needs the sport and triathlon needs Ironman.

The race is for sale now. It may already be a done deal. Whatever the case, I suspect that the future of Ironman is bright indeed. Any solid business deal has an element of human predictability involved. It is safe to say that for many years to come, there will be athletes from all walks of life who will want to do battle with their competitors, the element and themselves on a barren stretch of Kona coastline.

TRIATHLON MONSTERS–DEFEATING INTANGIBLE FEARS OF THE MIND

As a new parent watching a child grow, and taking part in your son's or daughter's new experiences, it's only natural to reflect on your own life and childhood years and try to remember how you felt about certain happenings. Nobody goes to school to learn this stuff, you just think about how your parents did it and either act in exactly the same manner or just the opposite.

Take monsters for instance. We all knew that they were right there under the bed, waiting for us to go to sleep before they reached out with those long slimy fingers and wasted us. But in the end, most people realize that the monsters weren't there at all, or at lest they take a different form now. Instead of two-headed giants, an adult monster creeps in the shape of fear, depression, insecurity and a host of other intangible beasts.

I used to think that sports training would enable anybody to conquer the creature in the dark closet. I don't know if I was right. Kids create monsters because of their fear of the unknown. When the lights go out, who's to say if the garbage they see on television won't come right out of the idiot box and swallow them alive. It is only with time and experience that kids of all ages begin to believe that they can control their environment and beat down the monsters of life. Physical challenges can present themselves from time to time, but are not always enjoyable or rewarding. You've got to throw down your own gauntlet from time to time.

Triathlon has its monsters, both real and imagined. The more tangible ones include sharks, cars, dogs and unseen holes in the trail. All of which can do harm to life and limb, if not screw up your whole day.

The first time I saw a shark in the ocean, I was a half-mile from shore on a surfboard. Each time you swim in the ocean you can bet that the "men in gray suits" are watching. The fact that they eat us less than we eat them is an incredible source of luck–don't you think?

While sharks and swimmers can safely co-exist in the same environment, cars and bikes cannot. When I leave the garage on my bike, motor vehicles become my natural enemy. Aggressive and irresponsible drivers will kill you and still be able to go to sleep that night. Don't ever forget that.

Finally, where a car is a constant and visible threat, a dog or a hole in the road that you twist an ankle in are the "sneak attack" monsters of running. Just when you were feeling comfortable and relaxed, you end up sprinting at a 4:30 mile pace as a Fido gains ground on you. This was an acceptable challenge until pit bulls became popular.

These kinds of monsters can be dealt with though; they're a known quantity that we all must face from time to time.

The ones that take place in our minds, not unlike those under the bed, take a different approach to overcome. I don't know how or why people develop fears and insecurities in life, but they do. I'm sure that it limits their potential to achieve the things that we call success.

That is one of the amazing things about endurance sports–they instill a tremendous sense of self confidence in those who partake in them. It doesn't matter how you do, only that you strive for and achieve some sense of control over your body, your mind, your destiny and the monster under the bed.

OBSESSION–SOME EXCESSES YOU CAN CULTIVATE

It never ceases to amaze me how society puts labels on us. No matter who or what you really are, if you follow a certain practice or act in a certain way, you immediately fall into an entire category, complete with label and typical psychological makeup. If you ride a motorcycle, you are a Hell's Angel. If you like mathematics, you are a nerd. If you live in the South, you are a Redneck.

We have all been stereotyped before, some more than others, but rarely does it happen that we are in a position to appreciate it. Usually, when someone prejudges us, it carries a negative connotation, and we react accordingly. But what, for instance, if somebody were to call you "obsessed" because of your undying penchant for endurance training? Would you take that as an affront to your mental stability? Obsession is not regarded as a normal trait. Or would you consider it a compliment that you are dedicated enough to your training that somebody would go so far as to put you in a category usually reserved for habits a bit less redeeming than exercise–like gambling or drinking?

Could it possibly be true though? Are you obsessed or, worse yet, addicted to exercise? Now, addiction is another word not often used in the healthiest of references. But there is the distinct possibility that you may in fact be addicted to your training. If you suffer from some type of depression when you cannot work out, it is a good sign that you are hooked. You can blame it on the lack of endorphin release you normally get or you can just say, "I needed to blow off some steam." Either way, you are a candidate for "Intervals Anonymous."

IA was formed to help people like you who can't seem to get in enough training yet fail to recognize or admit they have a problem. The first meeting I went to, I sat in the back and hid under a hat and Oakley sunglasses, trying desperately to avoid drawing any attention to myself. Gradually, though, I became more and more involved at the meetings until I was able to admit to myself that I was, in fact, a junkie. After several years and countless electroshock treatments, I can now discuss it in public and admit that I am hooked, I will never change and I am proud of it. Now when someone calls me "obsessed," I simply say, "Thank you very much. Have a nice day."

Intervals Anonymous is a tremendous organization. It is opening up chapters all over the world as more and more people come out of the closet–I mean locker.

If you feel guilty about missing that 20-mile run because you had to work in the yard, it is okay. I am here to tell you that you are normal. If you get pissed off when traffic forces you to be late for a swim work-out, you are not alone. I met a guy at an IA meeting who brought his wind trainer to his wife's hospital room while she was in labor. His condition is somewhat extreme, but hey, what if she was going to be there all day? Think about it.

If you feel that you may be affected, look for the nearest chapter of Intervals Anonymous and get some help today. Find out that it is okay to go to the track when your in-laws come over to dinner.

THE THRILL OF VICTORY–AT WHAT COST?

The great futurist George Orwell once said, "Competition is war without the gun." Indeed, countless examples support that claim. If you don't believe me, spend a Saturday evening at the bowling alley or a Sunday afternoon at the ballpark and watch the intensity with which men and women go at each other. And for what? For the rewards of victory, ranging from neighborhood bragging rights to World Series rings.

Competition is everywhere. It's part of human nature and has been since cavemen fought each other over the best caves. Competition has kept us sharp and inspired us to improve, and it has motivated us to kill each other over things like political ideas.

While most agree that competition is part of a healthy society, some of the various forms it takes are not. War is bad, of course. But are all sports good? And what of the relation between the two? Is there any? Or is Orwell's statement simply outrageous?

The need to compete exists in all of us to varying degrees, as does the need to succeed. The difference, however, is not often understood, and problems arise when the latter is much greater than the former. The pure, unadulterated act of competing can be a wonderful and healthy thing. But this is frequently overshadowed by the need to win, tainting the intrinsic benefits of testing oneself against others.

Much of the blame for this rests on our society. We pay baseball players more than presidents. We worship Olympic gold medalists and basketball players. I won't say they don't deserve reverence. But I sometimes feel that we have elevated sports to unhealthy levels of importance.

Consider the advice of Baron Pierre de Coubertin, the father of the modern Olympics. He professed that winning and losing are less important than taking part in the game. Compare that notion to Vince Lombardi's more contemporary view, displayed in his famous quote, "Winning isn't everything. It's the only thing." Lombardi, of course, was trying to motivate professional athletes to perform at their highest level. Still, this attitude often works its way down into contests with much less at stake than a Super Bowl title, and that is what's troubling.

We've all been to a company softball game in which something as trivial as a contested call at the plate festers into a raging argument with an umpire who, Monday through Friday, is the company warehouse manager. I'm not sure whether many of us notice this skewed attitude in ourselves. Such a loss of perspective has become acceptable under the guise of "striving for higher ideals" and "attaining our personal capabilities"; and unhealthy competitiveness is seldom recognized.

But who's to say when we're being overly competitive? One person's indifference to finishing a race first is someone else's laziness. For example, I don't consider myself competitive by nature. And I don't like to compare myself to others. Yet I have chosen a career in which I support a growing family by racing my heart out 20 weekends a year. It's a tough call.

I suppose the best for which we can hope is that individuals will use athletic competition not only as an outlet for aggression, but also as a means for self-discovery. We must not forget that the outcome has less value than the process.

A QUESTION OF BALANCE–WALKING THE TIGHT-ROPE BETWEEN EXTREMES

I stood poised, ready to make what could become the most famous–and the most dangerous–move ever performed at the Del Mar Regional Park. I balanced precariously on the end of the jungle gym's top rung, trying to ignore the children's requests to fly like Peter Pan, and breathlessly contemplated the challenge that lay before me: to walk along a two inch bar, suspended six feet off the ground, for–gasp!–about four feet. My mission was to reach the top section of the yellow and blue rocket ship, thereby becoming a hero in the eyes of the kids watching me from below. My other option was to climb down from this perch, dispensing lessons of safety, and summarily lose face in front of my daughter and the dozen other impressionable 5-year-olds. It was a weighty decision.

As a professional athlete, I am supposedly intensely aware of my fine-tuned physical abilities, knowing just how far I can push the performance envelope without going over the edge. But this was foreign ground to me. And in a moment of utter clarity, I realized that I was not only a weak excuse for a well-rounded athlete, but that triathlon was only a narrow manifestation of the science of cross-training. Any athlete with a sense of balance, average flexibility and adequate hand-eye coordination would have easily negotiated the jungle gym-to-rocket-ship leap.

But here I was, the great endurance guru, with an opportunity to achieve Evel Knievel-like stature among the members of the Torrey Pines Grade School Kindergarten class, and I was scared and wishing I could do something easy, like a 20-mile run. Triathlon is a wonderful sport for developing aerobic capacity, strength and endurance, but when it comes to balance, flexibility and coordination, forget it. (Have you ever seen a group of top triathletes playing basketball? After an hour, the score resembles that of a soccer game.)

The originators of the sport intended triathlon to involve those who could excel at several sports, and for many, swimming, cycling and running was enough. But now that most of us have gotten pretty good at those three, don't you think we should further explore the cross-training phenomenon and add a fourth or a fifth segment to our sport? How about tennis? That's popular. Or hunting? If we add hunting, we'll at least have something to barbecue while we wait for our age-group announcements at the awards ceremony. And do you think drafting would be a problem if we were allowed to carry guns on the bike?

Seriously, just because you ride 200 miles a week, don't think that you're entitled to some John Travolta-esque moves on the dance floor. The body adapts to the stresses we place on it, and if touch football isn't a regular occurrence for you, then all I can say is: Be careful.

Mark Allen's inability to sink a free throw is only one of this sport's interesting paradoxes. While long workouts strengthen the muscles and turn us into straight-line athletes, the drive to excel at triathlon has hidden costs. Many of us tout camaraderie in triathlon, the bonds we create through endurance training and competition. Yet those who spend exorbitant amounts of time in search of excellence must deal (or the people they know must deal) with the consequences of a self-centered athlete's lifestyle.

To do well, I mean really well, training has to encompass much of your waking day. If it's not swimming, cycling, running, weights, yoga or massage, it's eating, taking a nap or getting the gear ready for tomorrow. All of this comes at the expense of family and friends, employers and teachers. This is, of course, the extreme, but how many of us have made our husbands or wives drive to a race because we didn't want to waste any energy stepping on the brake pedal?

While balance may be the answer in most cases, it's still true that the more you put into it, regardless of the cost, the more you get out of it. As long as you recognize the costs and are willing to accept them, go for that extra-long ride at lunch. Who needs a job, anyway? You can always become a professional triathlete. It's a piece of cake–trust me. Just be prepared to do a good imitation of Olga Korbut on the playground so you don't wreck the image of pro triathletes–you know, that image I've worked so hard to build.

OF SKATEBOARDS, SPIDER WEBS AND SMILES

It's a curious fact that the worst work is always done with the best intentions, and that people are never so trivial as when they take themselves very seriously. Oscar Wilde, 1854-1900

I love my garage. Not only because I can organize it anyway I want, but because it's a sanctuary of sorts–a place I can escape to. It's a fairly typical garage in Southern California, only it's as crammed full of toys as it can be: surfboards, bikes, motorcycles, tennis rackets, basketballs, windsurfers–you name it. I rarely have time to use any of them, but the mere fact that they're here is somewhat comforting. The flagship of this fleet of recreational opportunities is an old skateboard that I've had since the earth was cooling.

For a variety of reasons, this plaything has come to symbolize my youth. Lots of older guys play tennis, ski and even surf, but few 35-year-olds come home from a hard day at the office and jump on his or her skateboard. In recent years, the skateboard has falsely come to be associated with rebellious urban teenagers. This only enhanced my affection toward an activity that I rarely partook in, but could still relate to.

My life took a turn one day, largely because of that skateboard. I had been too long in a state of constant stress from too many things happening at once: heavy training, overseas races, outside commitments, clothing company responsibilities, family, illness–you name it; shit was coming down all around me. I think they call it sensory overload.

Anyway, because of my peculiar zest for living, I was killing myself with things to do. I was learning that the nature of bright sunlight was to eventually cast long shadows. Along the way, I stopped smiling. And then I saw the skateboard. It was tucked away under the bench; the bearings were not only beginning to rust, but the tell-tale signs of non-use were clearly evident–spider webs. As I looked down at the dusty object, I realized that it was a sign–an omen of sorts that in my desire to take the world by the feet and shake the contents right out of its pockets, I was missing the point and forgetting how to laugh in the process.

It's easy to get caught up in society's guidelines for self-worth: material wealth, social and employment status, and political clout. For many years, I had shunned these, choosing instead to measure my self-satisfaction by health, lifestyle and the ability to ride my skateboard to the store for a quart of milk. And there I was, staring at my rusted symbol of freedom, realizing that I was no better than Joe Cholesterol down the street with his leased BMW. The biggest price I was paying was the loss of my happy-go-lucky approach.

I know that you can accomplish a lot and not fall into the trap–it's not easy, but if you have the right attitude, it's possible. I hadn't learned that attitude yet, and years later, I still struggle with the balance of responsibility and freedom. It was at that juncture, though, that I decided to downshift the momentum and try to get back the consciousness that provides peace of mind. For some people, it takes the untimely death of a loved one, and for others, a religious experience. For me, it was a dusty skateboard that started me on the road back to where I wanted to be.

You see, you can set your sights on the moon if you want and work your fingers to the bone to get there. Nothing is wrong with that. But along the way, you have to ask yourself why you're doing it and what the cost is–because nothing comes for free. If you make a million bucks, but lose your friends because you stepped on all of them getting to the top, are you really a rich man? Correct me if I'm wrong, but you can't take it with you when you go.

This whole thing has very little to do with triathlon, other than the fact that if we all had clearer pictures of why we trained and raced we'd probably win more–or at least we'd smile more. And isn't that winning?

LEARNING TO LOVE RUNNING–LISTENING TO YOUR HEARTBEAT

I feel sorry for big guys. Of course there was a time when I envied the tall, thick, large-muscled types, but that only lasted a few months, and I was eleven years old then. Everybody knows it doesn't matter what an eleven-year-old boy thinks. But now, as I finally begin to develop traces of compassion, I look at extra-large guys and gals, even if they're buffed, and can't help, but feel some strange, pitiful emotion. And it's all because they have to lug that extra mass around when they run.

In fact, most big folks don't really enjoy running for this very reason. But that's only my opinion, and other than last December when I gained five pounds, I weigh the same as I did in high school.

This isn't about big vs. small or thick vs. thin. Heaven knows I've been run down by a few guys toting an extra 15 or 20. It's about liking to run for no other damn reason than because it just feels good. To me, it seemed that when the "running boom" hit its peak in the early 80s, everyone was doing it for the most pragmatic reasons: "I need to lose weight"; "I'm getting ready for a big 5K or 10K (or fill in the blank)"; "I've got a bet with my neighbor"; "my doctor says I need to lower my blood pressure"; "I really look good in those little tight shorts, don't you think?"

All good reasons, of course. In fact, any reason short of committing a crime is probably fine so long as it gets you up and out the door. But simple altruistic motivation was rare. Still is. You just don't find many folks who will answer in all honesty, "cuz I like it," and then move on.

Can you learn to like it? Love it, even? Did you learn to like broccoli or sweet potatoes? Of course you can.

How about this one? Driving through the Midwest in the early 70s, I happened to be "jogging" along a rural country road. In a period of 30 minutes, three separate cars stopped and asked me, in this order, "Are you in trouble? Where did you break down? Do you need a lift?" This, of course, is not the time to explain to Mr. Haystack in his gun-racked pick-up that what he might consider torturous makes you feel good.

I must confess, though, I run for many different reasons. I run because I like to explore forbidden areas. If you're caught trespassing while running, you rarely go to jail. I like to run because when I finish I crack open a cold beer and put my feet up, it doesn't matter who is bombing who in countries I can't even pronounce. I need to run to stay one step ahead of my kids. One day, some teenager will come over asking about my daughter and will stare at her little, butt in jeans a moment too long, and I'll take him down on the garage floor and shake him up good. But that's what dads are for. And I'll do a better job of it if I run.

Maybe I'm preaching to the choir on this subject. Maybe all you tri-heads out there run for the most profound and lofty reasons. It doesn't really matter. It's just really neat to run across some old guy who's been at it for 20 odd years, not racing, not shedding pounds, not doing whatever his doctor says—just running, chasing his youth, delaying the inevitable when Sunday mornings don't bring crisp 15 milers, but sluggish 5Ks. All for no other reason than if he didn't run, well, he just wouldn't be the same guy.

I'M NOT A TRIATHLETE

For several years, I stopped calling myself a triathlete. At least for the purpose of avoiding tedious inquiries into how I could support myself on a bike seat or in a pool. I avoided the triathlete label quite often when I answered the perfunctory, "So, what do you do for a living?". If I told the truth, I had to follow it up with "And no, I'm not a trust-funder or a lottery winner either." So I became a fitness consultant or an apparel manufacturer or a writer.

The stereotypes that people generate are at best amusing and at worst falsely cruel. But that comes with the territory, so you have fun with it and play along from time to time. Once in awhile though, you have to take a step back and reaffirm that triathlon in general offers much more than the uninformed neophyte has come to believe. Yes, the races can be very difficult, but no, most participants are not masochistic. Why do we do it? How much time you got, bud?

And as for the sport lacking in refinement and culture, hold on a second. There are few mediums left in our modern society that allow men and women to work alongside each other, pursuing an individual yet common goal of excellence– where the real rewards are not fame and fortune, but personal fulfillment; where the competitive spirit is matched only by the depth of camaraderie at the finish line; where family and friends of the athletes will stand on the sideline with a sense of pride and wonder at what "their" athlete can accomplish; where simple acts of human struggle are played out willingly for the self-knowledge and confidence that comes with each personal victory.

And everywhere you look–from the compassion in the medical tent, to the smile on the winner's face–there is a sense of beauty. And if this scene is quite different from the image portrayed by a bad experience, so be it. If you look for pain and despair you'll find it–anywhere. But if you look for beauty and depth of human spirit, you will find that too. Only, in games of physical challenge, you don't have to look that hard.

LET'S GET REAL–STAYING GROUNDED IN A FLIGHTY WORLD

There are few things more laughable than reaching the answering machine of a pro triathlete and listening to some garbage about how he or she can't get to the phone because they are finishing up a set of thirty 100 meter repeats, butterfly on the 1:10 interval when you know damn well they're in the middle of a two-hour nap that was preceded by lunch and "Leave it to Beaver."

In fact, for some "Tri-Nazis" I know (a.k.a. Tri-Atollah, Tri-Klux-Klan) there is an accurate method for identifying their actual daily workout mileage–amount claimed divided by two equals real distance.

I like little formulas and word games like this. When you spend exorbitant time on a bicycle seat you often search for little things to occupy your mind. I once spent the majority of a 110-mile ride with my triathlete friend Murphy Reinschreiber trying to find another word in the English language that rivals "building" in its dual usage as a verb and a noun in the sentence. Terribly fascinating stuff.

Back to the point. In the sport of triathlon, as in life, things are not always as they appear. The other day I was reading a description of a particular race, and you would have thought it was the Second Coming! Come on folks, this is a sporting event, not the season finale of "Dallas."

It's important to dream, to shoot for the moon, but a healthy dose of realism helps ease the fall back to earth when the mission is over. If everything we've read about triathlons over the years were true, the following would be reality:

• There will be 220 million people competing in 30,000 triathlons around the world this summer.

• Finishing the Bud Light Ironman assures you a spot in heaven.

- Triathlon will be a premier event at the Olympic Games in Seoul this summer, and Dave Scott will represent the U.S.A. as athlete, coach, mechanic and dietician.
- Wetsuits will be allowed at all races this summer; but you must wear them the entire race.
- The Bud Light USTS will be producing events in 89 cities this summer; but still no permits for Orange County.

Triathlons tend to attract highly motivated, highly confident people. With that confidence comes some slight over-projection of fact at times. In most cases this is okay. If you look at many of the classic success stories, the individuals always seemed to live with one foot on experience and the other headed toward their dream. The balance is important, though. Finding that equilibrium can only come from paying the price of experience.

That cost can be high if your confidence/ability ratio is not yet in sync. Indy 500 winner Danny Sullivan once told me that in car racing, if you make a mistake at 230 m.p.h. they can't give you a ten yard penalty–you're already scorched hamburger. Indy is not a good place for the over-confident amateur. That would be like putting Lee Iacocca on the starting line of the World's Toughest Triathlon. He might have the proper mind set, but I'd recommend he put a few more miles on the bike.

This article is not meant to be negative in any way. I am merely providing an opposing viewpoint to some of the "Triathlon is Nirvana" material that you are constantly fed. Dreams and the illusions they encourage are healthy–if you keep one foot planted in reality.

Chapter 7

Can I Borrow Your Boots?

The people never give up their liberties, but under some delusion.
Edmund Burke, 1729-1797

Any fool can make a rule, and every fool will mind it.
Henry David Thoreau, 1817-1862

Sports is not supposed to be a metaphor for life's strivings, but it is. Every day. Young adults are not supposed to vent their anger and frustration on the gridirons and playing fields of the world, instead of in the back alleys. But they do. A Little League baseball team shouldn't have to be a prime vehicle for teaching community and camaraderie that should come more naturally. But they don't, and so it is.

Society shouldn't have to rely on the volunteer soccer coach or basketball league to provide leadership and opportunity for today's youth. But thank God these volunteers do.

Athletics allows us all–players and spectators–to experience the wonders, the joys and the tragedies of life in a controlled arena where the consequences are not life and death, but only varying degrees of victory or defeat. Sports gives us connection to our past when we learn the games of our fathers and our grandmothers. It also gives us the opportunity to feel the utter ebullience of a league championship or the depths of despair from a crushing defeat. And in between we are taught how to give, to take, to get along and to stand alone.

More than a metaphor, sports should be–and often is–a huge textbook about learning to live as a human being on the planet Earth. The only stipulation being that, to take the class, you have to play fair.

But the Earth is round–which often prevents a level playing field. Sports is, in fact, rife with the darker sides of life–cheating, dishonesty, collusion–you name it, and you'll find symptoms of deceit and treachery from the school yard to the International Olympic Committee. But, ironically, that's okay. The opportunity to combat these forces is itself a means to an education. As long as the fight is fair, the field level.

You see, on one hand you'll always have the soul athlete who, at his or her core, is motivated by such things as the desire for victory, the need for self-esteem and the simple love of physical movement itself. And you will always have people who are threatened by that personal power, who want to control the athlete and the game by regulation and by the pressures of media, money and power. While the common denominators between these two groups of people are ample enough to allow for professional relationships, the diametric opposition is such that win, win situations are rare.

The true greats, the legends of any sport, focus only on the task at hand: hitting a curve ball, making a three-point jumper, splitting the arrow. When your focus dissipates toward the periphery–the cheerleader, the fans, the score–you get eaten up and spit out.

In the end, you have to be faithful to your calling, align with others who share your passions, learn what you can from the game and from each other, and never trust a man in a blue blazer.

THE BUSINESS OF SPORT

Ask any 14-year-old what question he or she is most often asked, and it will probably be the ubiquitous "What do you want to be when you grow up? At least, that's what I was always asked.

Sometimes we can answer honestly; most of the time we lied to make our parents and teachers happy. We said that they had instilled wonderful values in us and we all hoped to become doctors and lawyers.

The truth is, at 14, nobody really knows which career he or she will end up in. But at one time or another, almost every kid who lived within ten miles of a playground dreamed of being a professional athlete.

Playing in the big leagues: *that* was the ultimate. No selling cars or having to fight the traffic–just hitting the ball or running down the field. And, best of all, you get paid for it.

It was, of course, just a dream. We all learned how hard it was to make it to "The Show," and society's guardians really didn't condone the pursuit of one's big-league fantasies past college graduation. Once you had a diploma in hand, it was time to "get on with your life." In other words, to do what everyone else was doing.

For a slim few with the talent, tenacity and fortune, the dream of professional sports became a reality. Whatever the season time for chasing fly balls or a quarter-finals berth in a tennis tournament–somebody, somewhere, was having his or her moment under the lights. The pros spend their workdays doing something the rest of the population paid to do on the weekend.

Along the way, sports became a business, a big business. Somebody figured out that people would pay to come out and watch the best play, to witness skill and thrilling competition. It was easy to see that spectators lived out their playground dreams vicariously through those down on the field. Of course they would pay to watch; they did back in the Roman Empire, and probably did before that.

At this point, cynics would claim duplicity. A true sportsman, it could be said, performs his craft for the purity of it. A paid professional is simply an entertainer.

The purist in me can empathize with this claim. Pragmatically speaking, we need people to reach the pinnacle in these various games. We need healthy entertainment, we need heroes, and well all know that given the chance to trade places for a moment—to run the bases after a solid drive to left field—we'd take it in a second.

I won't deny it. Business and sports are strange and diametric bedfellows at times. Even the words professional athlete form an oxymoron, like thundering silence, serious surfing or Elvis on CD. Athletes are, for the most part, inexperienced in the ways of business. And businessmen, as a group, don't understand the athlete's mind-set. This is a gross generalization, of course, but all you have to do is read the sports section of any major paper and the theory is given credence by the misguided dealings between professional athletes and the people who earn their living with the industry, but not on the field.

For some of the desk jockeys, the opportunity to pursue a career in a sporting related industry was the next best thing to actually playing. You are around people who like the same things you do, and you don't have the pressure to succeed in a limited number of years like the players do.

In some cases, executives are former athletes who decided to stay in the industry. Others however, simply found themselves treating one aspect of the sports industry like any other business. The fact is that many of the secrets of success in, say, the computer business, pertain to those of the tennis racket business or owning an NBA team. The common denominators in business of any type and athletics on any level are these: clear, concise goals; a willingness to follow your dreams; solid human values; dedication to the job; a deep desire to do your best and simple enjoyment of the process itself.

I know I've said it before, but I really believe that the true rewards are attained during any journey, not at the end of the trip.

I sat back in my chair—my mind drifting toward the subject of which wheels to use in the upcoming race—and half-listened to one of the other panelists answer a question from the audience. Doing several things simultaneously is a bad habit I picked up in the more-is-better decade of the 80s. (I was only able to break this heinous habit after a powerful moment of self-realization in which I found myself making dinner, talking on the phone, listening to the news and speaking to my wife all at the same time.) Anyway, I was shocked into the present by a question from a gentleman near the back. He wanted to know if there was any worry among the panelists, most of whom were professional triathletes, about having to get a "real job" one day.

It's odd, I thought, that so many people can't relate a profession like mine to other professions. It's as if the concept of professional athletics as a commercial enterprise has never occurred to them. For whatever reason—it could have been my involvement in Tinley Performancewear, or more likely because I was the oldest – I was handed the microphone and expected to answer.

I wanted to ask this guy if his concept of a "real job" was the same as most other people's—a job society deems normal and you define as boring. Instead, I tried to answer as diplomatically as possible. Yet his question underscored for me that most people identify sports with leisure time—something people do to escape the daily grind. They rarely stop to consider the many examples of businesses related to athletics, such as:

1. Sports as paid-for recreation. You pay to play golf; you pay for a fishing license; you even pay to park at some beaches. In most cases, the greenback you lay down goes into running the business, maintaining the facilities or simply creating the opportunity for you and others to return another day. Sure, to you it's merely enjoyment. But in most cases, if it weren't for someone's vested interest, you wouldn't have an opportunity to enjoy. It's like any other business.

2. Sport-equipment manufacturing. We all know that soccer without a ball is a little boring. The sporting goods industry is a billion-dollar-a-year enterprise in America alone. We love to play, but even more, we love to have all the toys. The industry that equips our sport, for example, employs thousands of people, many of whom have never run a step or swam 25 yards. The point is, manufacturing products for recreational use is big business.

3. Sports in health and medicine. An area often overlooked is the use of athletics as a means of healing, such as physical therapy, treating mental illness, and even augmenting social development. There are countless stories of kids who couldn't make it in the classroom, but went on to lead healthy and prosperous lives that contributed to society because their vehicle for growth was the playing field and not the work-place. Some critics say that sports in schools will detract from the purpose of education. But schools are meant to develop the individual as a whole, to prepare him or her to take a place in society and act responsibly. If that's accomplished through basketball instead of algebra, so be it.

4. Sports as entertainment. We all have a need for diversions, and no one can deny that sporting events are entertaining. The tickets we buy or the commercials we view on TV between innings all feed the engine that runs the business of sporting entertainment. The athletes who live out our dreams are part of that package—paid to do what most of us can't, giving us a thrill in the process. Sometimes, they even motivate us to get out and actually do it! The fact that they are often used a vehicles to help market products shouldn't detract from what happens when the world's best get together to strut their stuff.

I guess the greatest truth out of all this is that there is no difference between amateurism and professionalism. Behind any so-called amateur sport is a vast array of related enterprises–and individuals–that exists for profit.

Equipment, facilities, coaching, health workers and even the self-appointed national governing bodies rely on capital to provide a means for human beings to express themselves through physical movement.

At the root of the business activity, below the budget items, profit/loss statements and corporate flowcharts, is a bunch of grown-up boys and girls doing a refined version of what they once did on the playground.

ACCEPT THE RESPONSIBILITY

One thousand years from now, history will reveal that the 20th century was indeed a golden age for sports. If you consider that sports permeate all aspects of our society, from politics to economics to the very socialization of our children, it really is amazing. Entire sections of our vast communications network including newsprint, radio and television, devote large portions of their programming to coverage of college and professional sporting events. Not since the height of the Roman Empire, two thousand years ago, has such emphasis been placed on the simple act of physical games of contest.

But how simple is it, really? Professional sports for entertainment is a billion-dollar industry. Consider the relatively new field of sports marketing, whereby corporations of all sizes and types will use sports as marketing, promotional, and public relations tools to increase awareness or change the image of their products. The motive is increased sales and profits.

The Olympic Games have unfortunately become highly political. We have not had a boycott-free game in 16 years.

There may be some drawbacks to sport's influence in our society, but the positives outweigh the negatives. Sports contribute heavily to many children's development. It serves as a stress outlet for a sometimes tense work-force and gives millions of people around the world a tremendous sense of joy and accomplishment.

Because of all this, however, sports has become a vehicle of power. The most coordinated kid on the block becomes "King of the Playground." The elite professional having a great season becomes the object of fan adoration. Less visible people behind the scenes use sports to become power brokers–from little league coach to the league coordinator.

Triathlon is no different. There are several pockets of influence within our sport that control most aspects of triathlon. Until recently, the stakes weren't that high. Very few commercial activities were available within the sport until 1982. In short, people worked for free. Athletes, race directors, organizers, etc., were involved for non-monetary motives.

Some of that has changed. The financial opportunities now available have, on one hand, allowed a certain number of people to earn a living doing what they enjoy–staying involved with a sport they love. On the other hand, some of the innocence is lost, a victim of greed by those trying to make a fast buck. (Anyone remember the Diamond Triathlon of the Stars?)

There are basically six strategic groups that control triathlon.

1. The Athletes. The largest and ultimately most powerful are the triathletes. The age-group weekend warrior who trains and races for fun and fitness can, en masse, decide the future of the sport by supporting certain races or certain entities that follow below.

2. The Race Promoters and Directors. This group stages the production in which the rest of us are players. They line up the sponsors, gather the field, lay out the course and pray that, in the end, no one gets hurt. In the past, a few shoddy organizers have given this group a bad rap. In a lot of ways, race direction is the real endurance sport.

3. The Elite Athletes. The folks that win the races have a certain amount of control because many of them have been around for a while and have accepted the responsibilities thrust upon them. Better to control your own destiny than to leave it in the hands of others who you can't always trust. Who would know better than those in the trenches?

4. The Sponsors. Without the influx of corporate dollars, the sport of triathlon would stagnate in small-time mediocrity. Sure these guys use the association as a marketing tool, so what? The trickle-down effect from entities such as Anheuser-Busch enable the traffic cops to get paid on their day off so that the race is safer, so that no one gets hurt, so that... you get the idea.

5. The Media. Initially it was just a paragraph buried in the sports page. Now there are half a dozen "network time" slots, a slew of cable coverage, a glossy magazine and worldwide attention to the major races. The media controls what the rest of the world sees and thinks about triathlon. It's a heavy responsibility that can't be taken lightly.

6. Tri-Fed. The sport's national governing body has had its share of trials, tribulations, successes and failures. 1988 was indeed a tumultuous year for the organization. Whether it was greed, personality conflicts or a lack of communication, the bottom nearly fell out of a viable entity of our sport. Not good.

Which leads us back to group one–you. Take control of your sport. Don't let a behind-the-scenes power broker tell you what kind of spokes you have to use. If you accept the challenge to compete, accept the responsibility to contribute.

THIS DIRTY GAME–LET'S KEEP THE REINS IN A FEW CLEAN HANDS

If you go to Barcelona, Spain, next summer to watch the Olympics, and stay in an expensive hotel, you may see limousines pulling up and dropping off VIPs. As you stand in the lobby and wait to catch a glimpse of a world-famous athlete or two, you may be surprised to see exit the door a gentleman who is obviously (from his physique) not a track-and-field superstar.

No, this person is not an athlete, but he is connected to the Games in a way that gives him a large say in how they are run. He is a member of a sports federation, a national governing body, an international union or possibly a committee of one of these esteemed politically oriented groups. He has been sent to Barcelona to observe the Games as a delegate from his "constituency" and to mingle with a myriad other bureaucrats who, as a group, will meet and make policy for the thousands of Olympic athletes sitting in dorm rooms on the other side of town.

These men and women aren't directly involved in triathlon, but they know of it, and they will set the example for those who will come after them–those who will eventually decide the fate of triathlon.

As triathlon continues its maturation process and tries to gracefully shed its youthful peculiarities, we, the rank-and-file competitors, face a variety of decisions that will determine the look and feel of our sport well into the next century. Issues have come and issues have gone, but repeatedly the questions of government policy and distribution of power rise to the top. The vast majority of triathlon enthusiasts are somewhat apathetic, choosing to focus solely on training and day-to-day responsibilities. That's understandable. But, as in any organization, those who fail to voice an opinion must be willing to accept the decisions of those who take the time and energy to get involved and influence policy (whether they get paid for their contributions or not).

Triathlon is at a crossroads right now, yet most athletes don't realize it. Look around. You can feel the sport changing. Much of what the competitor sees and experiences at events remains positive and, in some ways, has improved. Races are safer now; they are well promoted and, in general, better organized. This has a lot to do with the efforts of governing bodies like Tri-Fed (which has finally emerged as the Good Guy).

But have we also lost something? Has the golden goose laid a rotten egg or two? In our frenzied rush to be accepted by the main-stream, to become a "viable sport" and attain the Olympic mantle, have we let our innocence slip away prematurely? Did we rush through the honeymoon thinking that a house in the suburbs would bring us the respect of our peers in other sports?

Along the way, we acquired a plethora of organizational "must-haves," including more rules, more government and more power in the hands of the people like our friend in the Barcelona limo. Everybody seems to want to use other sports as models for triathlon's growth. But why? We're different. Always have been.

Personally, I don't want triathlon to be like track and field or swimming or cycling. They set a poor example when it comes to bureaucracy. Track and field had an annual budget of $9 million in 1987; only 4.5 percent of that went to the athletes. Swimming worked on $4.5 million that year, of which $17,000 or 1.7 percent, went to the athletes. Sure, some of it trickled down through clinics, insurance, etc., but a large chunk stuck at the top, funding a league of desk jocks.

Headed Back

We certainly need strong support and representation at the national and international levels. But if triathlon is headed in the direction of, say, the Gymnastics Federation, which has 37 people on its board and more than 30 separate committees, and where less than one percent of a $6.9 million annual budget gets into the athletes' pockets, well, then

I'm headed back to Fiesta Island.

Fortunately, we aren't there. There are vehicles through which you can make yourself heard, and, believe me, you can make a difference. There are lots of fine people running this sport, but blind support for any old smooth-talker will ultimately lead to conflict and fragmentation.

When he was once asked about the politics in sport, Bela Karolyi, the famous gymnastics coach, said, "We must cut off the title hunters, the position hunters, the egomaniacs. Behind the honest struggle of our athletes, you will find a dirty game."

REAGAN, FORD TRUCKS AND JESUS AT THE 20-MILE MARK–THE POLITICS OF TRIATHLON

There is a battle brewing in the sport of triathlon. It's a relatively small, but escalating conflict and unknown to most of the triathlon population. But in its outcome is our sport's future.

Though this conflict retains soldiers who champion to both sides, the division is getting less gray and increasingly black and white. Like any conflict, if you cut away the rhetoric and grand-standing and eliminate the "just-cause" crap, you are left with a power struggle–a control contest. And the greater the price, the more intensely the battle is fought.

Now before I get accused of stereotyping and gross generalizations (or even of washing triathlon's dirty laundry in public), let me state that, yes, I admit that I'm over-simplifying a complex situation. But I do so from a neutral corner–at least for this article.

For purposes of discussion, we'll call side one the Red Team. The Red Team is organized, in fact they specialize in organization. They believe in the power of numbers, political process, decision by committee, Ronald Reagan, high school dress codes and a strict limit on the number of bananas each athlete gets at the finish line.

The Red Team despises professionalism (as it applies to professional athletes, that is) and believes that Tri-Fed, the ITU and the NRA are sacred institutions. Red Team members dream of an Olympic triathlon and think that the snickering, crybaby pros should wake up and get a real job. They think the sport is doing well, but would like to see more triathlons on TV. In summary, the Red Team is a tight-knit, grass-roots clan with slight bureaucratic overtones, a busy social calendar and a stiff fine for those who pay their dues late. They hold their annual meeting in Kona each October.

Team two, the Green Team, is not really a team, but a loose description of a certain individual. He or she is difficult to label because they don't belong to any group and rarely discuss their beliefs or intentions. They do, however, enjoy competition, limited camaraderie, long training rides and the freedom of an individual sport.

They believe in capitalism, Darwinism and could care less if the pros, juniors or volunteers make any money from the sport. They're in it for the personal challenge and expect people to follow the rules, but refuse to play judge and jury by taking the dream out of a competitor's heart and replacing it with a chin-strap violation.

Green Teamers are also bullish on the future of triathlon, but don't care about the Olympics or TV coverage because a lot of them don't have TVs. They drive Ford pickups, build their own bikes and have conversations with Jesus at the 20-mile mark of a marathon.

While there appears to be a fair amount of diametric opposition between the Red and the Green, some common values are prevalent. Both teams are resilient, proud and motivated. Both believe in the celebration of sports, yet exercise that right in diverse ways. While the Reds discuss swim splits after the finish, the Greens have a beer and listen to old Hendrix tapes.

Reds will exhibit traits of Green behavior, but Greens will only indulge in Red mannerisms to support a friendship. Each group has strong ties to endurance sports, but while a Red's philosophy of a sporting lifestyle centers on fair competition and group workouts, a Green can only profess a raw and primal desire to find his core self through personal challenge. It would not be true to say Tri-Fed and ITU are all Red. Nor would it be right to proclaim elite athletes Green.

This is not Socialism vs. McDonald vs. Mark Allen. It is not the lone wolf against the pack, but it is a contrasting view of how triathlon should grow in the future. The sport was born of unique, "never say die" individuals, but tell me the last time you saw Tom Warren or John

Dunbar in an official's meeting?

Growth necessitates restrictions. Otherwise, we'd all kill each other getting to the first buoy. But lose your faith in activity as a vehicle to achieve a desired lifestyle and... wham!... the motivation is gone and you search for a vehicle less congested, less restricted. (Witness the flattened growth of triathlon in America while mountain biking, in-line skating and outdoor trekking are booming.) Even Les McDonald, president of the International Triathlon Union, and a tireless promoter of Olympic status for triathlon, agrees. "My biggest fear," he once told me, "is that we'll get on the Olympic program, but the sport will have lost its steam."

The key to success in any battle is to not have one. If one side or one particular way of thinking eventually succeeds, in this case, both parties lose and the sport will wallow in anonymity that permeates such sports as broomball and Frisbee golf. What are the common denominators? Can an individual searching for his or her soul on the Queen K highway exist alongside the committee head discussing where to put the mile markers on the same highway? Like my friend Jimi said, "You don't have to join, you just have to believe."

PET PEEVES

Don't you hate it when...

- You've just wiped your hands clean before the swim start and roughed them up with sand so that they are more sensitive to the "feel of the water," and someone comes up to you and shakes your hand good luck with his slimy vaseline-soaked mitts.

- You're running in a pack of competitors and as you approach an aid station and reach out for a cup of water, the guy in front of you grabs it when he already has a cup in his other hand. So you grab the next cup, pour it over your head and realize you have given yourself a Coke shampoo.

- You're on the last few miles of a hard 90-mile bike ride, you're warming down, and some kid on a $50 ten-speed he got at the swap meet comes sprinting past you in high-top sneakers and Levis and looks back at you when he passes as if to say, "I kicked your, butt."

- The race organizer promised to have awards "any time now," so you hang around when you are tired and hungry, hoping to meet one of the famous pros and maybe win a prize in the drawing. But two hours later, you head to the car and hear over the PA system, "We are hoping to start the awards any time now."

- You wait an eternity for your chance to use the porta-john, and when you are finally at the front of the line, some guy slides in front of you, saying, "My wave is next, you don't mind, do you?"

- You run the whole race with the same guy right on your shoulder, and within ten yards of the finish he sprints ahead of you and throws his arms in the air like he's won the whole damn race or something.

- You finally get your picture in *Triathlete Magazine* and it's just out of focus enough that your buddies won't believe it's you.

- Your big toe-nail that finally grew back after six months appears to be headed for certain removal once again because you ran a marathon in shoes that were too small.

- You're so tired coming home from a race that you drive your car into the garage and forget that the bikes are on the roof rack... until you see a bent wheel come rolling down the hood of your car.

- You're trying to get to your transition area on a cold race morning and some over-zealous security volunteer looks at your beer belly and says the area is for competitors only. When he makes you take your sweats off and show him your numbered arms, you drop your new white T-shirt onto the greasy bike chain.
- Some guy at your office claims that if he could train full time, he would easily finished in the top ten at Ironman.
- Some punk kid no more than 14 years old keeps lapping you at the pool.

But, you know what really bothers me?

- When I go out for dinner at some fancy "nouveau cuisine" restaurant that takes reservations six weeks in advance, and then have two bowls of cereal when I get home because I'm still hungry.
- When a cycling traditionalist makes fun of my "tri-bars" and then goes out and gets a pair because Greg LeMond has some.
- When some guy comes up to me and says that he's read my book, seen my video, bought my clothing, has really admired my accomplishments and then turns to his wife and says, "Honey, meet the famous Dave Tinley."

Being able to find the humor in an irritating situation is half the battle, don't you think? For example, the other day I was on a long bike ride and stopped at a gas station to take a leak. The wall urinal was broken down, so I used the toilet. Not wanting to touch anything with my hands, I tried to flush the toilet handle—one of those stick kinds you just push down on—with my foot. Somehow, my Aerolite cleat found its way around the handle and locked into place. There I was, clamped in and ready to pedal the toilet away.

UNEASY BEDFELLOWS

In all of the ten years Tom Warren has competed in the Bud Light Ironman Triathlon, he's only been to the awards ceremony once. I find that interesting considering that he's been in the top ten overall four times and has won his age group another three. Tom thinks that the publicity and the recognition take away from his personal and individual accomplishments. Ironically, the media that Tom avoids would consider his attitude "good copy."

There is a picture hanging up in Toyota Triathlon Series race promoter Dave McGillivray's office of Jan Ripple finishing the 1987 Ironman. Ripple crossed the line in much the same state as Julie Moss during her famous baby-giraffe imitation of 1982. The picture shows that ABC was ready to record a scene that they had been trying to recapture for five years. Placing their cameras inches away from Jan as she courageously crawled the last few yards was disturbing. Jan was down on all fours with a 70 pound camera in her face, and Valerie Silk was trying to place the trademark lei around her neck.

It bothered me at first that this camera crew would be so bold as to infringe upon this woman's single greatest personal achievement. It reminded me about what a rock climber once said: "To reach the top is great–to have to tell someone about it ruins the experience."

But then I thought about the millions of people who will no doubt be inspired by this incredible scene when ABC's Wide World of Sports broadcasts its Ironman show. It often takes others' unique experiences, captured and portrayed by various forms of media, to motivate us to reach out for our own challenges. And therein lies the great irony of the sports/media relationship.

The sport of triathlon has been heavily affected by media from day one. It was Barry McDermott's classic story covering Tom Warren's victory in the 1979 Ironman in *Sports Illustrated* that sparked the fires that now burn in a million triathletes worldwide. The fuel was a desire inside these individuals to reach out and accept a new challenge–10Ks just didn't cut it anymore. But it took major network coverage of triathlons, sport-specific periodicals such as *Triathlete*, and constant pushing by race directors to get their results in the local papers to finally get the word out: "Hey, maybe there is something to this multi-sport madness."

The sports media were hesitant at first to leave the big three–basketball, baseball and football–to cover the "Big Four" and the rest of the "crazies" who supposedly "swam 112 miles, biked around Hawaii and ran up Mauna Kea." But, gradually, writers and journalists around the world saw that this sport could indeed provide some "good copy."

The conflict begins, though, when race promoters give the media carte blanche to do whatever they deem necessary to get their story. As the producer for ABC at last year's Ironman told a group of pros at a pre-race meeting: "We need to get in close to see the expressions on your face and to see you sweat." And that's okay, if it's done right, because to a certain extent, the future of the sport is dependent upon those TV contracts.

There are, however, lots of Tom Warren types out there who don't give a damn if they ever get their picture on the cover of the Rolling Stone–their involvement is more intimate, their goals personal. They view the media as distracting and disruptive.

Whatever the inequalities, the truth of the matter is that the media bring sponsors, who in turn keep entry fees down by providing an infusion of the corporate dollars that help fuel the growth of the sport. More growth means more and better races, more friends and more fun.

The sport has to set some guidelines, though. It has enough stature now to take a stand on the issues that include media involvement. The Ironman people don't have to let anybody who is creative enough to swindle a press pass get one (which, by the way, is relatively easy). Do you think Wimbledon lets 300 journalists sit courtside next to the players during the finals?

Meanwhile, all triathletes are probably going to have to deal with the media at some time or other, whether they realize it or not. It may be as simple as a truck full of photographers zooming by during your bike segment, or perhaps a reporter attempting to interview you as you're wincing with pain in the massage tent. Yeah, the media needs stories, and the copy is good for the sport. But that doesn't mean that you owe anyone anything. Feel free to tell a reporter to go to hell if he's an imposition.

One of the worst career moves I ever made was in snubbing Jim Lampley of ABC when he strong-armed me away from my wife into an interview before I was ready (after I'd just won the 1982 Ironman). But if it happened again tomorrow, I'd have to say I'd do the same thing.

Why I'm a Triathlete (or overcoming Little League failure)

When I was nine years old, my favorite book was Strange But True Baseball Stories. I thoroughly enjoyed the collection of off-the-wall tales about professional baseball–a sort of "Twilight Zone" for sporting enthusiasts. My favorite story was about a one-armed outfielder who had so compensated for his handicap that he was able to field, run and bat at the major-league level. I remember thinking that if this guy can make the majors with one arm, I should be able to make the starting lineup on my little league team.

I wasn't a starter that year; in fact, I warmed the bench for the guys who had what the coach called "advanced hand-eye coordination reflexes." Believe me, as a nine-year-old, not only did I not know what that was, I had no idea that sporting goods stores didn't sell it. All I knew was that I tried hard, went to practice, played in very few games and felt totally worthless when my family came to the ball park to watch our games, only to watch the neighbors' kids play.

During that year, two very distinct thoughts began to set in my mind. The first was that, given a choice, I would rather be responsible for myself and my own performance, and not have to rely on the whims of others–such as whether the coach was going to play his son in my position or not. Thus my gravitation towards individual sports.

Secondly, and most importantly, I began to realize that no matter what I did or where I went, there would almost certainly be someone just a little better than me. If I were going to be disappointed every time I didn't win the game or get the highest grade in class, I would live a life of constant frustration.

Every time I go to a race these days, I hear of people–pros and age groupers–talking in suicidal tones because they "lost." Everybody has a right to indulge themselves with self-pity, but I just can't see how anyone can feel bad about any race as long as three things happen:

1. You do the very best that you possibly can at that particular time.
2. You follow the rules and don't try to "get away with what you can."
3. The race organization does its job and allows you to concentrate on racing, and not on surviving.

Given these basic parameters–honesty, self-integrity and confidence in race organization–any competitor should be able to go out and do the absolute best he can, have a beer with friends at the end of it all, and go home feeling damn proud of himself. If he doesn't, then maybe he should stick to the bowling league.

Somewhere therein lies the secret to the phenomenal growth of the triathlon. For some reason, this sport offers a feeling of accomplishment and self-worth that doesn't come after a set of tennis or a round of golf. Maybe it's because the media have in some cases built the sport up to be larger-than-life.

Maybe it's the unique combination of the three events that provides those who compete in the sport with a bonus of self-validation. Or maybe it's just that those who are attracted to the triathlon are overly self-confident to begin with and find the sport only a medium for yet another challenge.

Whatever the reasons, these accomplishments should not be lessened by feelings of guilt over a less-than-stellar performance. You know if you've done your best. Who cares what anybody else thinks! Out of the entire population, anybody who even considers doing a triathlon is in the top one percent. Challenge yourself, but be proud of your accomplishments.

ME AND BOSTON BILLY

This is unreal. Here I am in Stratton, Vermont on the east coast of America, walking up a very steep hill. There is no trail, we bushwalk, following little pink ribbons that designate the route of this particular style of off-road running appropriately entitled a "scramble." It is six days after the Ironman, I have a raging cold and I constantly ask myself just what the hell I'm doing here, "scrambling" up the side of this mountain in 40 degree Fahrenheit weather. It is so cold that Kenny Souza has opted for his larger, jewel-covered bikini.

Nose running like a faucet, quads screaming, I glance over my shoulder and see my old friend, the marathon legend Bill Rodgers. He is competing in his first race of this type, unsure whether the raw, irreverent flavour of this event will leave him with enough energy for the more traditional 5 km he will race in tomorrow. "Bill," I ask, "How old are you now, 42, 43?" He grunts back "47" and then pulls away, grabbing Aspen trees for balance.

Both of us are way off the pace, fulfilling obligations, nursing maladies, saving it for another day. It's a poignant moment, really. Two grizzled veterans with a combined age almost four times that of the average competitors, not expecting to win, but participating for reasons that are many and complex. I thought about Bill, what must it be like to win the Boston Marathon four times? The New York Marathon four times? To be a world class runner for almost 20 years and now be walking up a boggy hillside with 200 other runners, most of whom have no idea of who he is, what his credentials are.

He is an anomaly. A man who will sit at a table at some podunk neighbourhood race and sign autographs for three hours, never feigning interest. Always the listener. But mostly, he is a runner.

As an elite athlete faces the inevitable performance decline that is commensurate with age, he or she must make decisions that affect "the rest of his life." You can always retire before the decline, rest on your laurels, and let the fans remember only the big ones. Or you can keep racing, modifying your goals, taking the good with the bad, slide into an age-group kind of a thing.

For professional reasons and because it gets harder and harder to stoke the fires, most top professional athletes choose the former. But Boston Billy is a runner, plain and simple. Not a glitzy made-for-TV pro that values cereal endorsements more than the gallant late career race effort that "only" puts him in the top ten.

He shakes his head as we crest the hill top and discover that the course now sends us up and down a slippery streambed, laced with moss covered rocks.

He could not be happy. He is not. The race tomorrow carries some weight; this trail run was supposed to be a casual warm-up jog. Obviously it is not–at any pace. But he is game. What the hell. Scrambles may be a big part of running in the next decade. He will adapt and though his 46 years will factor into his performance potential, he will run and he will compete for reasons that only he can know. And it is comforting to know that there are athletes who offer us hope, serving as role models for our young.

ORDER FORM

Trimarket

P.O. Box 60871-ST
Palo Alto, California 94306
USA

Phone: 1-415-494-1406
Fax: 1-415-494-1413

Payments must be drawn on a US bank. International orders, please submit an international money order drawn on a US bank.

Name: _____

Address: _____

Please send me the following:

_____ copies of finding the wheel's hub at $9.95

_____ copies of the total fitness log at $9.95

_____ copies of the total runner's almanac at $12.95

_____ copies of the total triathlon almanac at $16.95

In California, add 8.25% sales tax

Shipping, within USA $3.00 ($1.00 each additional)

Priority shipping, within USA $5.00 ($1.00 each additional)

Shipping, international air mail $9.00 ($5.00 each additional)

TOTAL _____

I understand that I may return any unused book for a full refund if not satisfied

finding the wheel's hub
by Scott Tinley

One of triathlon's enduring legends, the Ironman Hall of Famer tells it all in this his third book. Described by running's Bill Rodgers as "Scott Tinley brings you into the intense eye of the triathlon, spelling it out clearly and with a potent sense of humor. I found this a fascinating book."

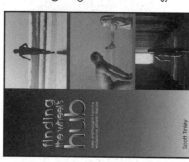

the total triathlon almanac

is the most detailed and comprehensive of all combined training logs and training handbooks. Specifically for the multisport athlete, this almanac is described by multiple Hawaii Ironman winner Mark Allen as, quote: "the best training manual and logbook on the market (and) Highly recommended."

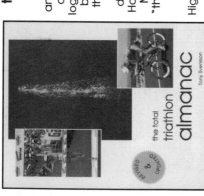

the total fitness log

this new multifitness book has advice from top fitness authorities. Includes sections on:

- cycling
- running
- walking
- nutrition
- swimming
- cross-training
- in-line skating
- mountain biking
- working out in the gym
- training with a heart rate monitor

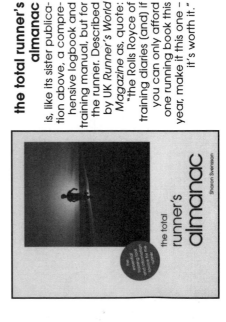

the total runner's almanac

is, like its sister publication above, a comprehensive logbook and training manual, but for the runner. Described by UK *Runner's World Magazine* as, quote: "the Rolls Royce of training diaries (and) if you can only afford one running book this year, make it this one – it's worth it."